SOAR: The Workbook
Achieving Your Best Possible
Health Through Awareness

By Dr. Roger White

authorHOUSE®

AuthorHouse™
1663 Liberty Drive
Bloomington, IN 47403
www.authorhouse.com
Phone: 1-800-839-8640

First published by AuthorHouse 1/14/2010

ISBN: 978-1-4490-1177-2 (sc)

Printed in the United States of America
Bloomington, Indiana

This book is printed on acid-free paper.

Notice

The self help health improvement program advocated in this book SOAR The Workbook is not meant to be a substitute for recommendations made by the reader's physician or health care providers. Each person has their own unique problems and needs and requires specific unique therapies that come from a partnership with their own healthcare providers. Maintaining this partnership is very important for effectual health care and should always be the cornerstone for anyone's total health care improvement.

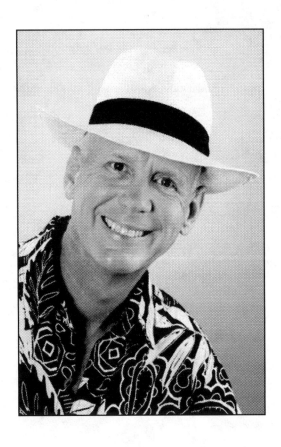

Dr. Roger White is a clinical cardiologist. He has been involved with emergency care, heart surgery, development of cardiac imaging, research, and teaching. He trained at the University of Chicago and has been on the faculties of Northwestern University Medical School and the University of Hawaii. He has published numerous scientific articles and a popular handbook for physicians on the modern treatment of heart attacks. He is a founding editor of the *Asian Annals of Cardiovascular and Thoracic Surgery* and is a frequent guest lecturer in both North America and Asia. He has made frequent appearances on television. His main interest now is preventive medical care. He coordinates lifestyle retreat programs in Hawaii and internationally. Dr. White resides in Honolulu, Hawaii.

DEDICATION

To my father and mother, Stanley White and Hazel Roll White,
for their gift of life and inspiration.

ACKNOWLEDGMENTS

Lynne Sandbach for her thoughtful and talented Illustrations

Emily Ann White (my wife), Natalie Reitman-White (my daughter), and Howard White (my older brother), for their continuous love, support, and advice.

Mary Jane Fainter for her reading review and comments.

Dr. John Klock, Cynthia Klock, Gwynn Williams, and Jeffrey Stone for their professional and personal support of me during my transition to preventive care.

The staff and editors at Author House for their excellent assistance in making this book a reality.

TABLE OF CONTENTS

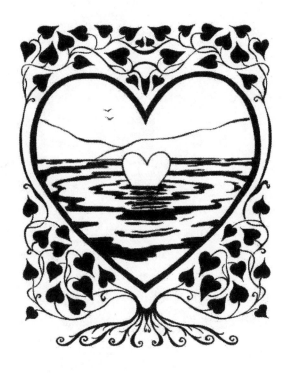

INTRODUCTION

SOAR guides you through questions and exercises in a workbook fashion to develop your own program for sustained total health improvement. Through awareness of your baseline physical and spiritual health, you will gain insight into your strengths and weaknesses and their interaction. Everyone is unique, but unfortunately, your health is ultimately determined by your weakest link. To improve your health, you need to identify your own potential weak links and develop your own specific plans for improvement.

There is a lot of dissatisfaction with medical care today. Mostly, this comes from inadequate or poor communication between doctors and patients. People's true and total needs are often not addressed, and both patients and doctors are discontented with the care rendered. They fail to work together as an effective team.

I developed the *SOARing Awareness Assessment* as a simple, low-cost, effective tool to help both you and your doctor enhance your awareness regarding your total baseline health. This includes not only your medical care, but your nutritional health, fitness level, and components of your spiritual health as measured by the quality of your relationships. The assessment is a tool to bridge the communication gap with your health care providers to make your visits more productive. Your doctor, if prudent, may even initiate this assessment, since it includes many items that have an impact on your medical care.

This assessment organizes all the components of your health in a systematic way. Often, when addressing health problems, weaknesses in your spiritual health are particularly neglected. These are things that your doctor may not traditionally evaluate. Ultimately, only you can improve these areas of your health. It is still important for your doctor to also be aware of your psychological stresses. Just know that you can improve your spiritual health, and its benefits are long-lasting. This will be the most important and rewarding component in improving your health.

The *SOARing Awareness Assessment* is just twenty-eight questions that I adapted from four-thousand-year-old universal health teachings passed down in many different traditions. I selected and modernized these questions to fit current times. The assessment follows the old teaching philosophy of asking questions to enhance your enlightenment. This way of teaching acknowledges that you already have the knowledge inside of you—it just needs to surface to your awareness. Asking a question just stimulates your awareness. To answer these twenty-eight questions honestly, you merely need to connect with your spiritual heart or consciousness and answer from your heart. The health assessment provided in the workbook is short and takes only about fifteen minutes to complete. It can be repeated frequently to follow your progress.

Each of the twenty-eight questions has a potential numerical point value, with the maximum score being 108 points. I purposely chose this number because I wanted something a bit more than 100 points. You could say that the number 108 is like SOARing (just a bit more than 100 percent). Think of it as a goal for continuous improvement, but understanding the journey to improved health is more important than an artificial destination.

I got the number 108 from my visits to Nepal; where there are 108 prayer wheels surrounding many of the temples. As these prayer wheels turn, they send messages of peace out to the universe. I was also once given a prayer necklace with 108 beads by a special spiritual leader. At one point in my life, I gave it to someone close to me as a prayer of protection during difficult times. I think that it helped. I do not really believe in numerology or talisman artifacts, but I do believe in spreading universal peace and good will at any opportunity.

Having a high or low score on your assessment is not important. A high score does not confer disease-free longevity, and a low score is not a death sentence. What is important is using your score to help you gain awareness so that you can take constructive corrective action.

You will tabulate your results in a blank *SOARing Awareness Graph*. Using this visual result, you will better understand your own results.

I am a cardiologist. I have been involved with many of the technological advances in cardiac care during my career; however, I have seen patients often remain ill in spite of advanced medical care or not recover because their total health was often neglected. As stated above, this is particularly true when problems in your spiritual health are neglected or ignored.

It is important to realize that you can still "SOAR" to excellent health in spite of any age or any current illness if you have two things. They are having an honest commitment to improve your health and secondly, forcing yourself to be truly aware of your potential problems that need correction. Only you can break your own passivity and "wake up."

If you deceive yourself, you will only limit your own progress. Everyone wants to be as healthy as possible; however, even if you have significant problems with your physical health, you can still lead an optimal life if your spiritual reserves are high. This is the secret of truly SOARing, regardless of age or medical condition. (Just remember numerous inspirational people like Helen Keller or Franklin Roosevelt that SOARed in spite of medical disabilities.) But to SOAR, you have to make a disciplined approach to improve your spiritual health every day.

Questions and exercises in this book will help you develop a disciplined approach to deal with your weaknesses. Most people have issues that they deny or neglect in their spiritual health that contribute to their health's decline. This may sound a bit non-medical, but as a cardiologist, I know that this is critically the most important thing to address when you are facing any physical illness.

Everyone, during his or her lifetime, will have physical and psychological traumas. Your physical health reserves, particularly in nutrition and fitness, need to be in place before an emergency to enhance your recovery. This is the essence of any preventative medicine program. But you must also remember that during any physical illness, your spiritual reserves are also challenged, and during any psychological crisis, your physical reserves are challenged. If your spiritual reserves, which are often overlooked, are not in place or depleted when acute physical illness strikes, your recovery with even the best medical therapy will be only temporary or incomplete. Chronic neglect or depletion of your spiritual reserves usually, in time, initiates physical illness. This book promotes a proactive, balanced approach to build up both your physical and spiritual reserves while you are still well so that you will be better able to deal with any future challenges.

There is a famous old saying:

"The only thing that is certain is change."

Passive change, whereby you just accept whatever comes along, is often destructive to your health. *The SOAR Total Health Improvement Program* encourages constructive, proactive, positive change. This puts you in the driver's seat.

To get the best improvement in your total health, you should review your results with your family. Families need to commit and improve their health habits together. In doing this, you will strengthen your heart to heart connections. Your plans are then more likely to succeed.

In your journey to improved physical and spiritual health, remember:

"Awareness without action is useless, and action without awareness is useless."

The *SOARing Awareness Assessment* is your first step towards creating sustainable change. Only you can stop doing harm and decide to change an unhealthy lifestyle. Only you can make the promise to do continuous improvement. Only you can connect to your spiritual heart or consciousness. If you do, then your spiritual heart will guide you in the right direction. This is because your spiritual heart always wants you to succeed. So enjoy the journey to your best possible health, and with insight and action, you will SOAR.

THE ACRONYM SOAR AND ITS PRINCIPLES

The Acronym SOAR and its Principles:

To help you take control of your health and SOAR, you need to understand all of the individual components that make up your total physical and spiritual health. If you see an eagle flying over the mountain, it has perfect balance and strength. It soars to new heights. You admire it and envy it. I use the acronym SOAR to help you remember these same principles of strength and balance when it comes to your health.

I believe that best possible health is based on four basic health principles. They are as follows:

S = **S**mart medical care
O = **O**ptimal nutrition
A = **A**ge-**A**ppropriate motion
R = **R**ich **R**elationships

A brief summary of each principle is described in bullet points below. The bullet point presentation here and elsewhere in this text organizes the material for your easy reference and review. Read each bullet point slowly and then pause for a few seconds and think how it relates to you. Make a mental note of areas where you may have weaknesses.

S = **S**mart Medical Care

- You really have just one choice when it comes to care of your physical health. That is: **Are you going to choose to *take care* of your physical health or not?** The Smart choice is obvious. That is why I used the adjective *Smart* and the letter S from this word to start the SOAR acronym. If you choose not to take care of yourself (by abusing your body, ignoring medical advice, not getting appropriate medical screening tests, or not taking prescribed medications), you are initiating your own decline in health. Taking active care of yourself will increase your probability of having good physical wellbeing. Active, positive participation is important for any medical care to be valuable. Therefore, start your improvement program by first making the Smart choice.

- Your physical and spiritual healths are absolutely interconnected and are always merging. When you receive medications or treatment, it is to address your physical health; however, it still concurrently impacts your spiritual health. Likewise, problems in your spiritual health, if uncorrected over time, will cause definite physical illness.

- When you need medical care, you want it to be competent, timely, and given to you with compassion. It is your responsibility to take advantage of the best that modern medical care has to offer.

- However, you need to understand both the benefits and limitations of modern medical care. Much more is known about the science of medicine than ever before; yet, physicians (and you) always work with incomplete knowledge. Also, advanced medical technology and treatment care may not always be available. Both you and your doctors need to always adjust to the best expertise, technology, and care that are available when you need them.

- Often, your doctor is in the position (particularly during an emergency) when he needs to act quickly to try to reverse your illness. Your doctor will never have all of the facts and will have to rely in part on his intuition. This is okay. Intuition is very powerful to help you determine desirable direction in life and comes from your spiritual heart. You can help your doctor by both giving him complete information about yourself and sharing your own intuition. This creates a more effectual partnership for your healthcare.

- A first-rate doctor will also appreciate your input that you may have regarding current medical knowledge. The internet has made the science of medical knowledge much more readily available. (Also, the internet has a lot of misinformation and half-truths.) You have much more time and vested interest to research your own medical problems than your doctor. Once again, only you can be hands-on and take accountability to understand medical concepts and potential treatments that are specific for you. When you partner with your doctor, you can share this knowledge. Your knowledge is modified by your doctor's expertise, and your doctor is exposed to different points of view that he may not have considered. Thereby, you arrive at joint decisions regarding your needed care. A prudent doctor will welcome this input, since their time to do research is limited by busy schedules. However, conscientious doctors are always willing to learn new things.

- Both you and your doctor need to be proactive in screening for illness and treating potential medical problems as early as possible.

- Reassurance of wellness is a fantastic medicine. You need to develop a trust in your doctor to overcome potential hypochondria. However, doctors must earn that trust with their expertise and compassionate care of you while always listening to you.

- When you are suffering illness, you want immediate reversal with treatment; however, patience is vital to recovery. Patience is an important part of healing. You need to maintain respect for your body, since it heals with its own timeframe. Treatments are received immediately, but you cannot accelerate healing. By being patient, you will be in accord with the way things are and achieve better results.

- Compassion, as previously stated, is the crucial ingredient for all care. Compassion is always available, but begins with you. Learn by heart that you get back what you give out.

O = Optimal Nutrition

- When you make daily choices of what you are going to eat, you need to concentrate more on **how you want to *feel* rather than what you want to eat.** If your nutrition is Optimal for growing, energy, and healing, you will feel better. I chose to emphasize the word *Optimal*, and that is why the letter O is the second letter in the acronym SOAR. Just like the other principles, it is equal in merit and always interconnected with the other principles.

- Nutrition strongly impacts your physical health. The old saying is "You are what you eat." True Optimal nutrition goes further, as it also strongly impacts your psychological and social wellbeing.

- I use the word *nutrition* specifically rather than the word *diet* because it is much more important than any diet. Fad diets (like weight loss diets) are temporary solutions that often depend on non-sustainable gimmicks. Sometimes, short-term diets can be helpful to achieve specific goals (like weight loss), but they are no substitute for a long-term sustainable approach to making healthy food choices. Good health is more important than just being thin. When you concentrate on your own specific nutritional needs, you adjust to change (which is inevitable). Practicing sound fundamental nutrition never stops working to improve your health, whatever your age or circumstance.

- Your focus when choosing food to eat should be that it is healthy. Eating healthy foods allows you to be energetic, grow, and heal. Therefore, making Optimal food choices is fairly simple. You simply choose to eat more foods that promote the above and fill up on these foods first. Filling up on the "good stuff" will reduce your hunger and help you avoid the "bad stuff."

- Healthy food choices include eating more organically-grown fruits and vegetables, having foods from whole grains, and eating more foods that contain "good" fats (Omega 3 fatty acids), like oils from flax seed or wild salmon.

- Next, you need to limit certain foods that in small amounts are okay, but in excess cause medical problems like obesity, diabetes, and high blood pressure. Food that contain excessive saturated fats (like dairy products and fried foods), refined carbohydrates (like sugar from desserts), and excessive salt (used in flavoring) should be limited. Learn better to steward small amounts of these foods in your diet.

- Lastly, you need to totally avoid, as best as you can, foods that have the potential to cause adverse health problems like heart attacks and cancer. These include foods that contain trans-fats (often present in food served at fast food restaurants), preservatives like nitrosamines (found in packaged luncheon meats and hot dogs), and cancer-causing hydrocarbons from highly smoked foods (like blackened, charcoal-broiled meats).

- The physical environment, in the form of plants and animals, becomes a part of you when you eat. Therefore, you need to help promote a healthy environment for both plants and animals and choose foods that originate from such environments to be part of your regular diet. That way, you will be healthier. Treat your immediate surroundings with gratefulness and compassion. This will come back to you as improved health.

- Nurture a spirit of gratefulness for everything you eat, recognize this, and share this with whomever you eat. Enjoy food in a social setting, and when preparing food, always do it with love.

<u>A</u> = <u>A</u>ge-<u>A</u>ppropriate Motion

- Everything that you do in your life involves some type of motion. **Consciously decide every day what you are going to *do* with your life.**

- Motion begins even before birth. It becomes more mindful and changes during your life. Motion is both physical and expressive. Physical motion attends to your more primitive needs. Expressive motion attends to your more evolved spiritual needs. Through both types of motion, you make many constant choices as to how you interact with the world and other people. Your choices involve how you work, play, articulate, interface with others, relax, and recover.

- Motion changes with <u>A</u>ge and needs to be <u>A</u>ppropriate for your specific situations. Age is part of your cycle in life and hopefully by learning from your experience, you gain wisdom with age. Also, your choices for both physical and expressive motion need to be <u>A</u>ppropriate to achieve the best possible results. I chose the letter <u>A</u> from both words <u>A</u>ge and <u>A</u>ppropriate to give emphasis in SO<u>A</u>R to what optimal motion is in life. Think of motion as everything physical and expressive that you do in life. As such it has a strong impact on your spiritual health. It is not just exercise.

- Motion is often considered physical condition, but ultimately, it is an expression of your inner spirit. Both physical and expressive motion reflects your actions for everyone to see. It shows the world who you are and is closely related to your spiritual expression.

- Regular physical exercise is an expression of your physical motion that helps you to maintain the best possible health. There is no such thing as anti-aging. However, regular physical exercise combined with judicious eating is the most important principle to slow your aging. It is better than any vitamins, creams, or facelifts! Not only does exercise give you better appearance, it allows you to enjoy your advanced years with less disability. This belief is important to remember each day to motivate you to do regular physical exercise.

- As you get older or have a medical disability, do not concentrate on what you cannot do, but concentrate on what you can do. Stop comparing yourself to others. Just do your best, and you will know have that satisfaction. When you adjust to situations, you can still live life to its greatest potential. Being creative and adjusting are the keys to success.

- If either your physical health or spiritual health (or both) are severely challenged, a disciplined program of improving fitness through exercise and combining this with good nutrition will build your physical confidence, which in turn will allow you better to deal with your medical or spiritual problems. This is fundamental, whether it be recovery from physical problems like heart attacks or cancer or psychological problems like lack of self-worth or addiction.

- Obesity has become a common health problem. The emphasis needs to be on fitness rather than fatness. Everyone has the potential to be fit, no matter what their physical size. People genetically come in many different sizes, and everyone should respect this diversity. If you concentrate on physical fitness, your body will find the shape that it was meant to be. Size does not change who you are.

- You need to understand the elementary physical law of motion that states that wherever there is action, there is reaction. This means you also need balance physical exercise with rest and relaxation. You heal when you are sleeping. Make the right setting for good quality sleep. Appropriate rest and nurturing of your body facilitate good health.

- This above-stated law of physical motion is even more important in influencing the quality of your relationships. You need to balance receiving with giving, reflection with action, calmness with passion, listening with talking. If you are always giving, acting, or talking, you deprive yourself of true interaction. You become incomplete. When you actively are aware, you purposely seek a balance of the above symbiotic attributes. This will definitely improve the quality of your relationships. This involves all physical and expressive interactions, and especially true for sexual expression. True intimacy is one of your greatest expressions in life. This is only achieved by both giving and receiving.

- Whatever you choose to do in life, do it with passion and you will be healthier. In this way, you will always be respected.

<u>R</u> = <u>R</u>ich Relationships

- You are going to have relationships in life with yourself, others, your ancestors, and a higher spirit, whether you want it or not, so why not make them <u>R</u>ich? **Choose every day who you want to *be*.** It is through all of these relationships that you will understand your role in life. This understanding starts with understanding of yourself. All of the above relationships are continuous, synchronized, and interdependent. When you choose to make all of your relationships <u>R</u>ich, you promote good total health. Destructive relationships will always challenge your health. That is why I chose the adjective *rich* to emphasize choosing <u>R</u>ich Relationships and use the letter <u>R</u> to complete the acronym SOA<u>R</u>.

- Relationships are the cornerstone to your spiritual health. It is also easier to objectively evaluate than the concept of spirituality, which is somewhat vague and personal. When relationships (with yourself, others, your ancestors, or a higher spirit) are destructive, this instigates illness. In fact, this is often a more common precipitator of illness than even a decline in physical health. Its decline is usually more insidious and pernicious. This disruption is often unrecognized during illness, when both you and your doctor tend to focus solely on restoration of your physical health.

- If your spiritual health is diminished, either from lack of self-worth or because you are experiencing an abusive relationship, this will eventually cause physical illness. Your total health will never be restored unless all components of your spiritual health are addressed.

- Healthy relationships take time to develop but are the longest-lasting component of your four principals of most advantageous health. Likewise, broken relationships take a long time to heal. Healing of broken relationships is similar to healing after a heart attack. With a heart attack, you receive treatment and healing starts. Healing then proceeds on its own schedule. Healing of broken relationships does not start until there is mutual forgiveness initiated as a treatment. Healing of the relationship will not be immediate after the forgiveness is exchanged. It merely allows healing to begin.

- One of the most important broken relationships that you will ever heal is a broken relationship with yourself. Everyone has this at some point in his or her life. Search for insight to forgive yourself and allow healing to begin. When you cultivate rich relationships and forgive, you overcome other physical health problems when stressed. Improving all of your relationships deserves your full attention and should always be one of your top priorities for improvement.

- You need to make time and create the right setting to improve all of your relationships (with self, others, and a higher spirit). You have to stop multi-tasking and focus solely and soulfully on this priority. You cannot intently listen if you are not fully engaged.

- Spend regular time appreciating nature, as this provides the right setting to experience rich relationships.

- You also need to be aware of things that influence your life that have been negative psychologically handed down to you. I call these negative *trans-generational behaviors*. These psychological influences can be very harmful if you are unaware of them. You can feel ill at ease for unknown reasons related to your inherited psychological stresses. These can go back many generations, and you may not have the information to clearly understand their origin.

- Psychological influences from your parents (or surrogate parents) are especially strong and may have a negative impact on your day-to-day life because of something that happened years before you were born to them. Being aware of these influences is the first step to changing negativity in your own life.

- If you find psychological negativity in your psychological ancestry, do not blame them; just accept it and use it to build your own character with your consciousness. You always have the capacity to break negative trans-generational behaviors. Remember, too, that you are a model for behavior if you have children. Children pick up more on what you model, rather than what you say.

- Keep your language pure and impeccable so as to be an exemplar for your child and others. Your language reflects your soul for all to observe. Also, be cognizant of your moods and actions, as these will be reproduced in your children. Think about things that may be negative in your personality that you psychologically inherited. Be aware, so that you do not replicate these behaviors and dispositions in your children.

- You also need to avoid both gossip and assumptions (most of which are false). Both of these are toxins created in your mind that usually have adverse consequences for your relationships. Be aware and identify gossip and assumptions and try your best to avoid them. Stop assumptions or gossip earlier before they become destructive.

- Relationships come and go in life and have different purposes. Embrace all of them and respect them for what they are. Bless past relationships. All relationships are mysterious because they are both constant and changing (even with persons who are dead, since your perspective of the present is always influencing your past recognitions); however, all relationships start with you. Be grateful for who you are. Always remember that you are unique and worthy. All life is interconnected.

- Everyone is of equal merit. Life is always changing. Embrace change and change with it. Do not think that your actions are superior or isolated. If you are searching for a mate, try to be the right type of person, rather than trying to find the right person. You will be more successful and maintain your self-worth.

- In dealing with people, try to pay it forward. This is a popular phase and philosophy based on looking for opportunities where you can help people unconditionally and proactively. Your actions with one person may impact many other people at a later time. Each time you do something positive for someone, it can have a cascading positive effect.

- Your greatest legacy in life will be the quality of your relationships. The true importance of a legacy is purposely nurturing relationships while you are alive. A legacy is not so much something to leave behind as it is a daily goal to live by. Actively think about what you want your legacy to be with those closest to you. Remember this and live proactively and accordingly.

The Stability of Your Health is Like Standing on a Chair with Four Legs

For your physical and spiritual health to SOAR, you need these four principles of health to be strong; but you are only as healthy as your weakest link.

To illustrate the interaction of the four health principles, imagine a chair with four legs that you want to stand upon to reach something that is above your natural height.

- You need those four legs on that chair to be strong and balanced if you are going to safely stand on it. If any leg is weak or out of balance, you will lose your balance and fall. The strength and balance of the total chair are only as strong as its weakest leg. Before you stand on that chair, you need to heighten your awareness to be sure that it will support and balance you. If a leg is weak or out of balance, you need to proactively correct this deficiency before trying to stand on that chair. Only by doing that will you successfully stand on it with confidence and reach your goal.

- With guidance from your spiritual heart or consciousness, you can balance the four principles (SOAR) like four legs on a chair to achieve the best possible health, but this is only achieved through dynamic awareness combined with remedial positive actions.

- Your awareness of the strength and balance of the legs of the above chair can be misinterpreted through your arrogance. You may think that you just need three strong legs to stand on that four-legged chair. You ignore one weak or imbalanced leg. Because you are arrogant, you think that you can overcome this weakness without correcting it because your other three legs are strong. This chair with a weak leg supports you only for a while; however, arrogant thinking causes you to ignore the strength and balance of the total chair. If you inadvertently shift your weight towards the weak leg when you need it, the chair breaks and you fall. Your arrogance caused your fall. So it is with your health.

- Arrogance comes from the brain and is an illusion. You do not need it to survive. It is a toxin to the body, just like ungratefulness and hatred. Arrogance comes from an inflated ego, which comes from a sense of insecurity. Arrogance frequently precedes illness. It is easy to see egotism in others, but harder to see it in yourself. If you are overconfident, people have little empathy for you when you fall. They say, "He was heading for a fall."

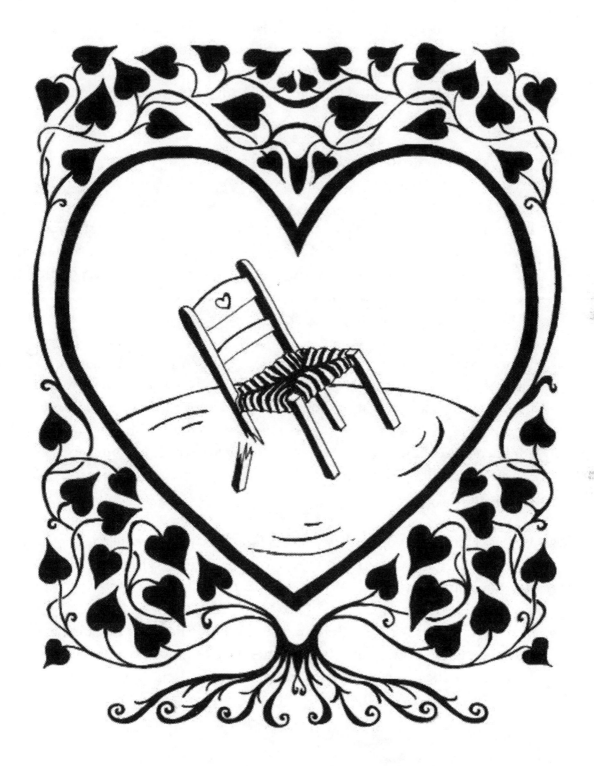

In summary:

- Your physical health and spiritual health are on a continuum and not separate. Physical medicine, nutrition, motion, and relationships combine to determine the quality of your health. They can objectively be evaluated, and areas of weakness can be identified and improved through awareness. This will be done with the *SOARing Awareness Assessment*.

- Your physical health determines the quantity of your life. Your spiritual health determines the quality of your life.

- Physical and spiritual health is not separated! Each strongly influences the other. Strength in one can improve strength in the other, and weakness in one can cause weakness in the other. Always try to improve your weakest link first and at the same time, build up and maintain reserves in other areas of your health for when they are needed during an emergency.

- Improvements in your spiritual health may be the most challenging because only you can correct it. You may also be fixed in adverse habitual patterns that limit your insight and improvement. This is where discipline and improving physical health through good nutrition and exercise can build the physical confidence to allow you to deal with problems which are often related to unworthiness. If spiritual difficulties remain uncorrected, this leads to self-destruction.

- Everyone during his or her lifetime will face stresses and challenges regarding both physical and spiritual health. It is your choice to become a victim or develop character when faced with adversity.

- You cannot choose your battles, but you can choose how you are going to fight them. Cultivating awareness, being in the present moment, and facing issues honestly are the first steps towards winning any battle.

THE SOARING AWARENESS ASSESSMENT

BE STILL AND KNOW

To have insight, you need to be still and feel connected to a greater energy. Your spiritual health declines when you are excessively busy. When you are constantly busy, your mind overrides your heart. Your busyness causes numbness, just like the effects of too much alcohol. You fall into a trance.

The only way to break this trance is to be still, and to listen to the knowledge that is already in your spiritual heart. This is the oldest of many universal spiritual teachings.

There is a very wise saying, as follows: "Be still and know that I am" (adapted from Exodus 3:14 and Psalms 46).

When I have been working late at night at the hospital in difficult emergency situations, I have often felt stressed and even questioned my abilities. I never knew what I would be facing in the emergency room. What if I could not help the patient? I would often initially feel anxious or inadequate.

That was the very time I needed to remember the above advice. To remember it, I would just pause for a second; take in a deep breath and then exhale, and then just "be still" for a second before seeing the patient. I would ask my heart for direction. Inevitably, I would receive the right direction. I was grateful for this direction. This would calm me and prepare me to deal with the patient's emergency. At that second of recognition and calmness, I knew that my spiritual heart, the patient, and a higher spirit were all one and connected. This would help me as best as I could to give the patient a favorable outcome. By being still and accessing my spiritual heart, I could better adjust to the unknown. I could stay fully in the present moment.

This was the most important and practical lesson that I learned in my medical career and life; yet, even I frequently forget it! This is because my own busyness from my brain is in constant battle with the wisdom from my spiritual heart. This is when I need to recognize my own anxieties and limitations and get back to the basics of being still.

If you are ready to just be still, you are ready to take your assessment.

The SOARing Awareness Assessment

Read each question below and then pause briefly before answering. Be truthful and let the answer come from your heart. Do not think too much about each question. This assessment is only of value to you. There is no need to try to achieve a high score. Breaking your own trance and gaining your own awareness are what is important.

This assessment is not static, but will actively change as you change. With awareness, you can make change positive and assertive. Cultivating awareness and creating positive change on a daily basis are the goals of this assessment. There is a blank summary sheet at the end of this section to tabulate your results and draw your results on a graph.

Smart Medical Care Questions

On questions 1-6, score as follows (use summary sheet at the back of this section):

Score 1: I feel weak in this area and definitely need help.
Score 2: I feel okay, but could definitely use improvement.
Score 3: I feel good in this area, but know that I can improve.
Score 4: I feel great in this area, and I am SOARing.

- Question 1: How do you feel about your overall physical health?

- Question 2: Do you have a good understanding of how your body works?

- Question 3: Are you proactive in taking charge of your health? Have you had a recent good checkup with appropriate screening tests?

- Question 4: Do you avoid things you know to cause bad health, like smoking, excessive alcohol, inappropriate use of prescription or non-prescription medications, etc.?

- Question 5: Do you have a good partnership with your medical caretakers? Do they treat your whole health? Do you understand the benefits and limitations of your medical care?

- Question 6: Are you truly grateful for good health, and do you acknowledge this regularly?

Question #7 in this area has a different score system, as below. This question requires a sincere, honest reply from your heart.

- Question 7: What really is your desire to take better care of yourself every day?

Score 1: I know that I have deficiencies, but I really don't want to change.
Score 2: I want to improve, as long as it is convenient and does not take too much work.
Score 3: I am really committed to make necessary changes to maintain and improve my health. I want to SOAR in this area.

Optimal Nutrition Questions

On questions 8-13, score as follows:

Score 1: I feel weak in this area and definitely need help.
Score 2: I feel okay, but could definitely use improvement.
Score 3: I feel good in this area, but know that I can improve.
Score 4: I feel really great, and I am SOARing in this area.

- Question 8: How do you feel about your overall nutritional status, weight, and energy level?

- Question 9: Do you understand basic principles of good nutrition and how they apply to you?

- Question 10: Do you eat a lot of healthy foods like whole grains, fruits, vegetables, good-quality protein, and good types of fats, which include omega 3 fatty acids? Do you limit excessive caloric intake?

- Question 11: Do you limit foods that have excessive refined carbohydrates, saturated fats, salt, alcohol, and caffeine?

- Question 12: Do you actively avoid foods that are harmful to your health, like foods that contain trans-fats, chemicals, highly smoked foods, and foods that are high in nitrates, chemicals, and preservatives?

- Question 13: Do you enjoy most of your meals with friends and family and demonstrate your gratefulness at mealtime?

On question #14, there is a different scoring system similar to question #7.

- Question 14: What really is your desire to make real changes to improve your overall nutrition and feel better every day?

Score 1: I know that I have deficiencies, but I really don't want to change.
Score 2: I want to improve, as long as it is convenient and doesn't take too much work.
Score 3: I am really committed to make necessary changes to maintain and improve my nutritional health and SOAR.

Age-Appropriate Motion Questions

On questions 15-20, score as follows:

Score 1: I feel weak in this area and definitely need help.
Score 2: I feel okay, but could definitely use improvement.
Score 3: I feel good in this area, but know that I can improve.
Score 4: I feel really great in this area, and I am SOARing.

- Question 15: How do you feel about your body, endurance, strength, flexibility, appearance, and energy level relative to your age and condition?

- Question16: Do you understand the basics of physical fitness and training and what is appropriate for you?

- Question 17: Do you do regular aerobic exercise (walking, running, swimming, bicycling, etc.) at least four times per week for at least forty-five minutes?

- Question18: Do you do regular strength training and flexibility exercise at least three times per week?

- Question 19: Do you naturally sleep well and feel rejuvenated? Do you take time every week to nurture your body with massage, sauna, stream, or Jacuzzi therapy?

- Question 20: Are you able to balance both giving and receiving in your relationships? Do you give and receive in your intimate relationships?

Again, question 21 has a different scoring system, like questions 7 and 14:

- Question 21: What really is your desire to do things better in your life every day?

Score 1: I know that I have deficiencies, but I really don't want to change.
Score 2: I want to improve, as long as it is convenient and does not take too much work.
Score 3: I am really committed to make necessary changes to maintain and improve my health. I want to SOAR in this area.

RICH RELATIONSHIPS QUESTIONS

On questions 22-27, score as follows:

Score 1: I feel weak in this area and definitely need help.
Score 2: I feel okay, but could definitely use improvement.
Score 3: I feel good in this area, but know that I can improve.
Score 4: I feel really great in this area, and I am SOARing.

- Question 22: Do you feel worthy?

- Question 23: Are you the type of person you would want to be around? Are you happy, self-confident, calm, reassuring, and positive towards others?

- Question 24: Do you really treat others as you would like to be treated?

- Question 25: Are you able to freely express your feelings and emotions, and are you able to listen to others express their feelings and emotions?

- Question 26: Do you believe in a higher spirit, and have you felt it working in your life?

- Question 27: Do you balance your reflection with actions, and are you grateful for everything that happens to you, whether it is good or bad?

Question 28 has a different scoring system.

- Question 28: Are your actions consistent with the type of person you want to be every day? If you were to die today, what really would be the legacy of your relationships with yourself, others, and a higher spirit?

Score 1: I know that I have deficiencies, but I really don't want to change.
Score 2: I want to improve, as long as it is convenient and does not take too much work.
Score 3: I am really committed to make necessary changes to maintain and improve my health. I want to SOAR in this area.

You have now completed the assessment. Tabulate your results below and draw in your results on your *SOARing Awareness Graph.*
Next, you will need to formulate action plans to improve your areas of weakness.

Blank SOARing Awareness Assessment Summary:

Circle your score and then add up total points

Smart Medical Care Questions

Question 1: Score 1 2 3 4
Question 2: Score 1 2 3 4
Question 3: Score 1 2 3 4
Question 4: Score 1 2 3 4
Question 5: Score 1 2 3 4
Question 6: Score 1 2 3 4
Question 7: Score 1 2 3
Add up total score in this area _____

Optimal Nutrition Questions

Question 8: 1 2 3 4
Question 9: 1 2 3 4
Question 10: 1 2 3 4
Question 11: 1 2 3 4
Question 12: 1 2 3 4
Question 13: 1 2 3 4
Question 14: 1 2 3
Add up total score in this area _____

Age-Appropriate Motion Questions

Question 15: 1 2 3 4
Question 16: 1 2 3 4
Question 17: 1 2 3 4
Question 18: 1 2 3 4
Question 19: 1 2 3 4
Question 20: 1 2 3 4
Question 21: 1 2 3
Add up total score for this area _____

RICH RELATIONSHIP QUESTIONS

Question 22: 1 2 3 4
Question 23: 1 2 3 4
Question 24: 1 2 3 4
Question 25: 1 2 3 4
Question 26: 1 2 3 4
Question 27: 1 2 3 4
Question 28: 1 2 3
Add up total score for this area _____

With a marking pen, draw in your own SOARing graph, using the scores from the previous questions.

My total score in **Smart Medical Care** is _____. Mark and color this in bar over letter S.

My total score in **Optimal Nutrition** is _____. Mark and color this in bar over letter O.

My total score in **Age-Appropriate Motion** is _____. Mark and color in bar over letter A.

My total score in **Rich Relationships** is _____. Mark and color in bar over letter R.

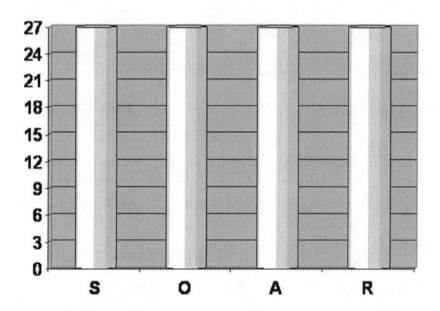

MY SOARing AWARENESS GRAPH
DATE_____

GRAPHS FOR FUTURE ASSESSMENTS

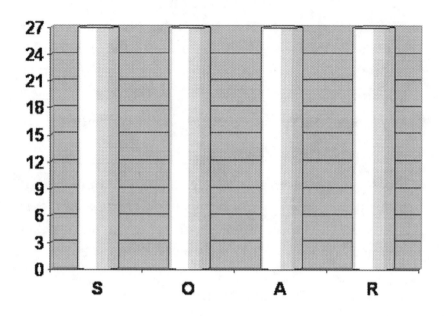

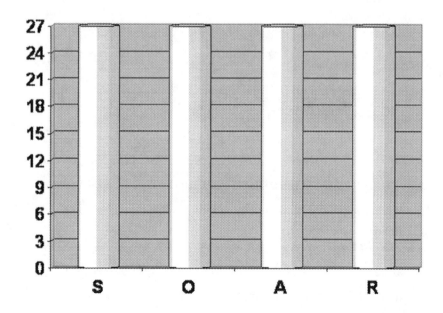

Understanding Your *SOARing* Awareness Graph

After you have completed the *SOARing Awareness Assessment* and have drawn your results with a dark pen on a provided on a blank *SOARing Awareness Graph*, you need to understand and reflect on your results before you decide on corrective actions.

You can see how each principle impacts the others by looking at your own *SOARing Awareness Graph* chart.

The graph below is an ideal bar graph chart summarizing the four components of your health (SOAR, as previously discussed). This graph is not from a patient. It is graph with a theoretical perfect score. It is to show you how to read the various bars on the graph so as to assist you with your own interpretation of your results.

The vertical axis has a total point score of 27 points. Each bar has a potential for 27 points, and the total of all four graphs is 108 points.

The horizontal axis contains the letters from the previously mentioned acronym SOAR to distinguish each of the four areas of your physical and spiritual health. Below is a key to remember the abbreviations on the chart from the acronym SOAR.

<u>**S**</u> = <u>**S**</u>mart medical care
<u>**O**</u> = <u>**O**</u>ptimal nutrition
<u>**A**</u> = <u>**A**</u>ge-<u>**A**</u>ppropriate motion
<u>**R**</u> = <u>**R**</u>ich <u>**R**</u>elationships

The sample graph below is a theoretical perfect SOARing score, 108 out of 108, with each of the four areas at its maximum score in total balance. The perfect score of 108 is merely an objective and never should be considered a destination. When you color in your own graph, most likely you will have some high bars and some lower bars. This is fine. This is true life! However, since your ultimate health is determined by your lowest bar, you should concentrate on improving this area first, while at the same time maintaining those areas that you are strong in.

Below this sample bar graph are additional descriptions with symbols: > (which means greater) and < (which means lesser). These symbols show the relative influences as you scan your bars from left to right.

Key to graph abbreviations:
<u>S</u> = <u>S</u>mart medical care
<u>O</u> = <u>O</u>ptimal nutrition
<u>A</u> = <u>A</u>ge-<u>A</u>ppropriate motion
<u>R</u> = <u>R</u>ich <u>R</u>elationships

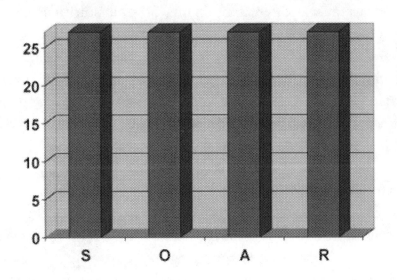

> Physical Health   > Spiritual Health

< Less Control   > More Control

< Fewer Choices   > More Choices

< More Transient   > Longer lasting

- As you review the *SOARing Assessment Graph*, bars to the left, you will see the letters (<u>S</u>) for <u>S</u>mart medical care and (O) for <u>O</u>ptimal nutrition. These areas reflect greater components of your physical health. With physical health, you have less control and fewer choices, and it can be very transient. Physical health is more primitive than spiritual health, but still very much needed for optimal function.

- Much of your physical health is determined automatically (called *homeostasis,* or autonomic function) and determined by your genetic makeup, age, and environmental exposure. You need to make wise choices to make your physical health as good as possible. This involves taking advantage of modern medical advances and eating healthy foods; however, you also have to accept a certain amount of fate. Illness happens; deal with it.

- Below the bars to the right of the *SOARing Assessment Graph*, you will see the letters (<u>A</u>) for <u>A</u>ge-<u>A</u>ppropriate motion and (<u>R</u>) for <u>R</u>ich <u>R</u>elationships. These areas reflect greater components of your spiritual health. Here you have much greater control over your destiny. You have many more choices. Improvements in spiritual health are longer lasting. Your spiritual health is more highly evolved. It requires your active participation to improve, much more than your physical health. You can choose to enrich this part of your life or waste it and self-destruct. In other words, "Don't waste your wonderful life."

- Your *Soaring Assessment Graph* is merely a snapshot of your current health. It is always changing. You will always be subject to external, passive change which you have no control over. The purpose of the *SOARing Awareness Assessment* is to heighten your awareness regarding the four components of your health so that you can make active change in those areas where you do have power to control your destiny and improve your health to the best possible and make the most of your precious life. You can still SOAR even if you have advanced age or serious illness. In fact, this is the very time when you need the most awareness and commitment to make the most of what you have.

MEDICATIONS FROM YOUR SPIRITUAL HEART

The Power of Mini-Meditation (HEART)

Before you get started with any effective change, you need to focus your attention. Meditation is very helpful to focus your attention. You can connect to your spiritual heart or consciousness anytime in a very private way. I did this myself in the previous discussion about being still so as to help patients better in the emergency room. I formalized this mini-meditation and use an acronym, HEART, to help you remember its components. Mini-meditation is particularly helpful during worrying times, when you may not know which direction to take. To mini-meditate do as follows:

- Stop, or Halt, doing what you are doing for a few seconds. It is vital to mindfully stop so that you break the cycle of your anxiety. This transitions you to be in what is called the present moment.

- Next, Engage and Experience what is happening right now. Continue to experience and breathe in slowly. Take in few deep breaths and feel your lungs expand. Meditatively breathing in and out quickly reduces your adrenaline level and creates mindfulness.

- Ask for guidance. When you are humble, you become receptive to input. Your spiritual heart or consciousness responds better to humility rather than arrogance.

- Once you access your spiritual heart or consciousness, you will Receive the answers that are right for you.

- After you have received your insight, give Thanks. This creates a cycle of respect that will perpetuate your actions and make them sustainable.

The above can be remembered as the acronym HEART:

- H Halt
- E Engage and Experience
- A Ask
- R Receive
- T Thanks

- Practicing this mini-HEART meditation just takes a few seconds, but it has tremendous benefit in preparing and focusing your actions. You will ultimately be more effective with your time. You will partner with all of the wisdom that your spiritual heart contains because it connects to an omnipotent energy. That wisdom is infinite and will guide you to the right action that creates inner peace. Peace of heart gives peace of mind. You can and should do this several times per day.

- Don't wait until you have a major crisis to practice HEART. Do it frequently, even for small things. When you become proficient using HEART for small problems, you will be better able to do this when you face more major problems. Asking for guidance will make you healthier and costs nothing. It is the most valuable tool that you have to improve your health and guide your actions.

- When you practice HEART, no one will know that you are doing these mini-meditations. However, people will know that your actions are more mindful. This is what it means to trust in the spirit of your heart, and with its all-knowing wisdom, it will always guide you to what is best. This will allow you to make heart-to-heart connections with others and a higher spirit when you need help.

AWARENESS EXERCISE

Create the right setting for contemplation and change. Spend some quality time by yourself in reflection without distractions. Go for a long walk in a beautiful place. Leave your cell phone behind. Breathe in and breathe out and connect with yourself. Feel alive and appreciate life. When you feel alive in every cell of your body, make a commitment to achieve your best possible health, regardless of your age or any underlying current medical disabilities. Practice the above HEART meditation when faced with daily stresses and choices in life. Use it when driving in heavy, frustrating traffic, rather than some obscene gesture. If it's right for you, combine the HEART meditation by putting your hands together in prayer, closing your eyes, and kneeling down. This can facilitate your meditation.

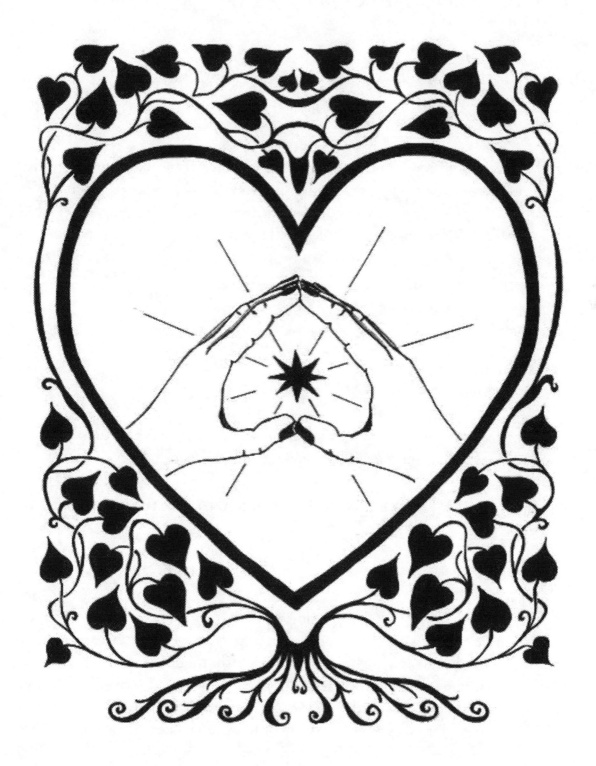

Medications that Come from Your Spiritual Heart that You Need to Access Every Day to Help You SOAR

There are medications that you put in your body to help it function better, like blood pressure medication, cholesterol-lowering medications, blood thinners, and vasodilators.

There are even more important medications that come from within your spiritual heart or consciousness that promote good health and healing. They are in endless supply, even in people who may not have accessed them in a long time. These spiritual medicines are always available and have no adverse side effects: however, they will never be expressed unless you make a conscious choice to access them. These medicines are as follows:

- Gratefulness
- Compassion
- Humility
- Forgiveness

You do not need to wait to start healing and improving your health. When you access these medicines today, you start immediately to improve your health.

Start Every Day with Gratefulness and Compassion

These are two of the most important medicines that reside in your spiritual heart or consciousness.

- Being grateful just takes little time to reflect and break your trance. You just need to say "Thank you" and appreciate whatever you have, rather than what you do not have. This applies to health, food, accomplishments, and particularly relationships. However, for gratefulness to become real, it must be demonstrated. You need to take time to acknowledge your appreciation for everything. This takes just a few seconds to once again briefly halt and let this recognition come from your heart. You need to recognize and appreciate both small and large things and things perceived as both good and bad.

- Acknowledging gratitude for bad things in your life can be very difficult. Reflect about things in your own life that you thought of as bad that in time turned out to be good. Everyone has such experiences. Also, during difficult times, try to bear in mind that things that are perceived as bad at the moment have potential to build your long-term character. This can help you get through complicated times.

- Unfortunately, gratefulness is practiced less and less in our fast-paced, high-achieving societies. If you neglect gratefulness, this becomes a toxin. As with all toxins, you need to be aware and totally avoid them if you want to be healthier. No amount of good deeds will overcome intermittent toxic ingratitude. When you are ungrateful, you view yourself as a victim, your self-worth will diminish, and your health will always deteriorate.

- Likewise, compassion begins with how you feel about yourself. This dramatically influences how you feel about others. The cycle of both giving and receiving compassion is just like the cycle of breathing. To live, you need to both breathe in and exhale. To experience compassion, you need to both give and allow others to give to you their compassionate gifts.

- Think of your compassion like a large lake that receives water and gives off many streams. If the lake never receives water (compassion), it will be empty and dry up into a desert. It will be unable to create streams. If the lake holds on to water (compassion), the plants downstream never get nurtured, and the lake becomes stagnant or dead. Allow your lake to both fill up and give off and flow freely with compassion. Remember, *you* have the power to start the cycle of compassion with unconditional giving. At some point, in some way, compassion that is given will always come back to you.

It is very important to first focus on *being kind to yourself.* This was the title of a series of interviews that I gave for a television series filmed in India many years ago on how to prevent heart attacks. The most important thing that came out of the television series was to remember, "You were born worthy." Worthiness and compassion and health are interlinked. No one can take worthiness away from you, except you. If you are feeling unworthy, the best way to reconnect to your worthiness is through simple, compassionate actions towards yourself and others. Remember that everyone else is also worthy. This will decrease your hatred, which is created in your mind. This is another toxin to your health. In simple words, "Hate less, and love more." This will create a sustainable cycle that is certain to improve your health.

- Like gratefulness, compassion only becomes real by doing compassionate actions. Good intentions mean nothing. It is only your actions that count. You need to ask yourself each day if your actions are consistent with the type of person you really want to be. In other words, if you want to *be* compassionate, you need to actively and consciously *do* compassionate actions.

- The great paradox is that compassionate actions towards others, although difficult during times of stress, will create the above cycle that will restore your own self-worthiness and health. First, concentrate on doing little actions with great passion, today!

Now, write your responses to the following questions:

GRATEFULNESS EVALUATION

- How have I recently demonstrated my gratefulness for my health, food, and relationships?

- Could I have been more grateful?

- What toxins (ingratitude) can I eliminate today?

- What am I going to do today to be more grateful?

COMPASSION EVALUATION

- How have I recently been kind to myself and others?

- Could I have been more kind to myself and others?

- What toxins (hate) am I going to eliminate today?

- What little acts am I going to do today with great passion to be more compassionate?

HUMILITY SETS THE STAGE FOR HEALING

When you access humility from your spiritual heart or consciousness, you better maintain awareness. Humility will help you survive life much better than arrogance. You are better able to identify your weak links.

- To establish a habit of humility, you need to be aware of when you are arrogant and reduce its presence. Remember your self-worth and be secure with that fact. You need to feel secure and self-confident and avoid pumped-up egotism, which is a mental aphrodisiac toxin. Understand that when you practice arrogance, it will ultimately be self-destructive.

- Actively choose to humble yourself. If you do not humble yourself, most likely at some point, you will be humbled. Once again, realize how great life is. Also, realize that life is not centered on you.

- Humility promotes empathy, which is important for heart-to-heart connections. These heart-to-heart connections improve the quality of your life and responsiveness. This will make you healthier. If you are humble, when you have problems, people will want to help you

When you cultivate your humility, you will feel better immediately. Now, reflect on these questions so as to create your own action plans for improvement.

Humility Evaluation

- What are recent experiences where I have been arrogant or humble?

- Was I more successful in accomplishing what I wanted by being arrogant or humble?

- How can I reduce my arrogance today?

- How could I have been more humble today?

- What am I going to do to be more humble today?

Forgiveness of Self and Others is the Strongest Medicine to Heal Yourself

Lack of forgiveness is the biggest impairment to best possible health. People hold back forgiveness when instead; it should flow freely and continuously, like your circulation. Failing to forgive is like holding onto a red-hot piece of coal with your hands. By refusing to let go, you only hurt yourself. Let it go, and let healing begin.

- This is easier said than done. The main reason for lack of forgiveness is your brain saying that you are right. Right or wrong has nothing to do with forgiveness. Judgment is your viewpoint. Extending forgiveness does not mean you forget or condone bad actions. When you give forgiveness, it needs to be sincere and avoid anger or blaming. It needs to be as immediate as possible and unconditional. The biggest benefit of forgiveness is that it allows you to begin your healing and not be a prisoner of the past.

- People frequently create physical health problems because they do not forgive themselves. Something happens in their past that they just cannot get out of their minds. It may even be the result of a negative trans-generational behavior that has been passed on to them unknowingly. This is common with violent and abusive behaviors. The end result of lack of forgiveness is feeling lack of worth. This is where trying to get to the root cause of your lack of forgiveness is very important. When you have that "light bulb going on moment" of awareness, you are then ready to drop the hot coals that are burning your soul.

- If problems of self-forgiveness seem insurmountable, here again, professional help may be needed to break through barriers. Professional consultation may take the form of a doctor or psychologist, a pastor or priest, or just a trusted, wise friend. Restoration of total self-worth and self-forgiveness are reciprocal.

Like previous medicines from your spiritual heart, you need to access this every day. Practice forgiving little problems every day so that you are experienced in forgiving when bigger problems come.

Review these questions and write your responses so that you remember them. Share them with needed people involved and take action.

FORGIVENESS EVALUATION

- Is there something that is causing me to make myself ill because I do not forgive myself?

- Can I recognize this and begin to forgive myself today so as to let healing begin?

- Is there someone that I need to forgive?

- How can I forgive this person so as to facilitate my own healing?

- If someone has forgiven me, have I recognized this and helped them with their healing?

MAKING MINDFUL CHOICES TO IMPROVE YOUR HEALTH

How You Make Mindful Choices to Improve Your Health

As stated earlier, if you are aware but do not act on that awareness with constructive actions, it is useless. It is like touching a hot plate and being aware of the pain, but not letting go. Once you have taken your assessment, you will need to formulate action plans to improve your weak areas. To do this, first you need to understand the difference between back-ended medical care and front-ended medical care, and how it relates to your wellbeing.

Back-ended medical care is reactive, or crisis-oriented. Everyone requires this type of care at some point in his or her life. Back-ended medical care is initiated by symptoms of illness. Your illness gets diagnosed, and you seek competent medical care. The problem with this type of care is that it only treats un-wellness and often does not get to the root of many people's problems.

The goal of back-ended medical care is to restore health and return you to your baseline. The problem is returning to a baseline that often involves an unhealthy lifestyle. This, as previously mentioned, results in reoccurrence of illness. Recurrence of illness can be prevented through gaining insights and education.

Everyone has a certain amount of denial that illness will happen to him or her. You think that you can get away with something like avoiding exercise, overeating, or even beginning to smoke. You feel that you are young, different, or blessed. You rationalize your benefits. These are false rationalizations. It is better for your health to recognize these rationalizations as false early and avoid their associated harmful behaviors so as to reduce health problems at a later stage in life.

DEALING WITH ADDICTIVE BEHAVIOR

- The absolute worst behavior is doing something you know is harmful for your health, but you just keep doing it. This is the basis for addictions. Addictions to excessive alcohol and drugs are obvious. They numb your awareness and thereby cause your physical and spiritual health to deteriorate.

- Other, less obvious addictions to bad speech, anger, sex, vanity, and work are more subtle but have equally dangerous consequences for health over time. Basically, all addictive behaviors are the result of a gradual loss of self-worth. Whatever the addiction, you think that it gives a temporary reappraisal to deal with your problems; however, when the temporary numbness wears off, your pain from the problem causing the addiction is only worse. Addictions create a downward spiral that is certain to end in illness.

- Everyone is prone to addictive behaviors. This is the biggest cause for self-destructive illness. Recognize this and be aware of what your addictions are.

In the space below, write down your addictions so that they come into your consciousness. Think about the obvious ones and the less obvious ones. Ask people close to you what they think your addictions are. Are you hiding things from others?

ADDICTION EVALUATION

These are my small addictions:

These are my major destructive addictions:

These are what other people think my addictions are:

Do I really want to change my addictive behaviors?

CREATING AWARENESS WHILE YOU ARE WELL IS IMPORTANT

Awareness and desire for corrective action come very quickly when you are sick.

Unfortunately, during a medical crisis, your treatment options are often limited. I have treated many patients with acute heart attacks. They came to the emergency room because they had new and intense chest pains. Their pains made them very aware that something was wrong. However, by the time they had a heart attack, the disease process was advanced, and my treatment options were often only palliative. This is true of most diseases that are diagnosed during an emergency.

I would prefer to intervene earlier in the patient's care to totally prevent the heart attack. This could be done by encouraging healthy lifestyles, getting appropriate screening tests to detect early heart disease, and starting corrective therapy before there is heart damage. The problem is that it is difficult to initiate this type of change when you are feeling well. When you are feeling well, you are often unaware and see no need to change.

Palliative care received during a health crisis can still be life-saving but is definitely associated with increased disability. Furthermore, crisis-oriented care also costs you precious time, which can never be replaced.

BENEFITS OF FRONT-ENDED MEDICAL CARE

You can see that what I recommend is mostly *front-ended medical care*, which is preventative and proactive. Front-ended medical care involves frequently evaluating your baseline health to make necessary, continuous corrections and improvements. When you practice preventive care with a healthy lifestyle, you will build up your health reserves. This can both prevent illness and reduce the impact of unexpected illness. This is best done *before* there is a crisis, when you are feeling well. You have to be continuously aware and make an effort to store up your health reserves for when you need them during a crisis.

The ultimate goal of preventive care is always to totally prevent illness and maintain wellness. When you identify weaknesses early, then is the time to make the necessary changes so as to avoid catastrophic illness. This takes commitment, education, and sustainable actions. This involves the partnership with your doctor that I addressed earlier. Preventive care is not easy but results in much less long-term disability. If practiced, it will ultimately give you more quality time in your life. One of the key principles with front-ended medical care is that the earlier the positive lifestyle adjustments are made, the bigger and longer the impact will be on your subsequent health.

Could you be more proactive in monitoring your medical health? If so what do you need to do? Write you responses below:

Maintaining Your Health Over a Lifetime Is Like Flying a Spaceship to the Moon

Here is a simple way to remember the importance of early corrective change to stay on course with your health. To further understand this important principle of how early intervention impacts your health; pretend that your health is like flying a space rocket to the moon.

- Flying a spaceship to the moon and back is a long and complex journey. The course of the journey is never perfect. Your health over a lifetime is like this journey. The spaceship always needs continuous adjustments to stay on course. Small changes made early in the direction of the spaceship's flight will determine whether it is on the right course to reach the moon. A seemingly minute error in direction early in the flight, if not corrected, will result in the spaceship missing the moon by thousands of miles later in the journey. A small adjustment that could have been made early in the flight to stay on course becomes a very large and costly adjustment later on in the flight.

- So it is with your health. You may not always make the right corrective decision, but if you are aware, you will self-correct faster. For example, a small correction to lower your cholesterol and have regular exercise at age forty (or earlier) may prevent that heart attack in the middle of the night at age sixty-five or sooner. But just like navigating the spaceship to the moon, maintaining your health takes many active decisions to go in the right direction. The longer you drift off-course, the greater your likelihood is for severe illness or premature death.

- To stay on course, you need to feel your entire body working together. Every part of your body relies on the other parts for performance and must be respected. It is just like an orchestra playing together and in tune.

The good news is that even if you have neglected your health for years, it is never too late to improve your health. As you age, your risk for heart disease, stroke, cancer, arthritis, and degenerative neurological disease increases. This can make aging depressing! Good health is harder to maintain the older you get. Age is part of the cycle of life, but you can live optimally at any age or in any situation. The best way to stay on course is to make early, instantaneous adjustments. Making simple, positive changes anytime in your life improves your health and reduces your need for crisis-oriented medical care. You can even do this when you are ninety years old and frail, but still live life with vigor

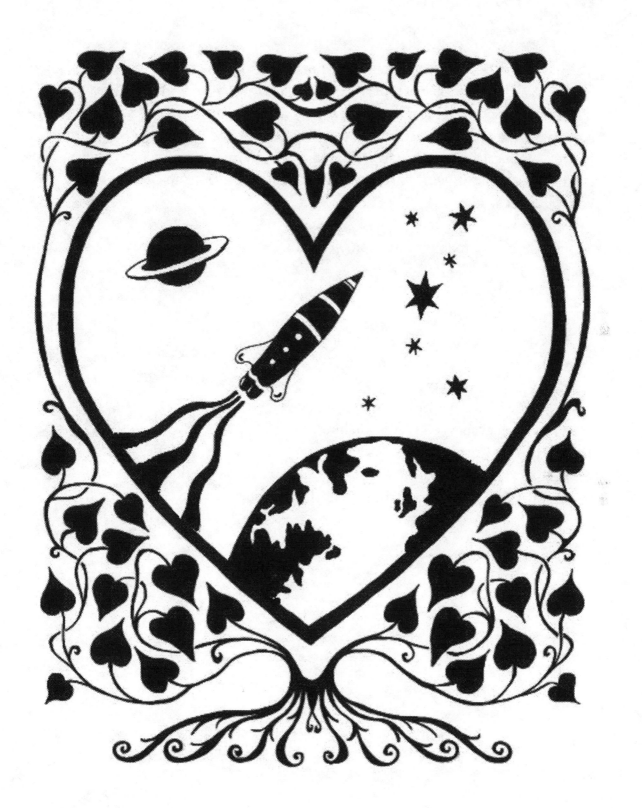

Effective Change

You have now prepared your heart to evaluate and improve each of your own areas of SOAR. What follows is brief material on each area of SOAR and some examples of recommended action plans. You will need to develop your own specific action plans. Make your plans achievable, but not too easy. Share your goals with family members, friends, and health care providers. Set tentative target dates for achievement, but do not become compulsive. Adjust your plans as needed. But most importantly, make your changes sustainable.

To introduce the following sections, remember these points if you truly want to change:

- Commit to change with a passion.
- Become aware of your baseline.
- Be in the present moment.
- Establish a plan for change.
- Set achievable goals and timelines.
- Execute the plan.
- Reevaluate and adjust plans as needed, based on results.
- Sustain actions over time so that they become fixed in your heart.

STEP ONE:
IMPROVING YOUR PHYSICAL HEALTH

STEP ONE:

IMPROVING YOUR PHYSICAL HEALTH

The acronym below (CARE) is added to help you remember the key recommendations to improve your physical health.

Acronym: **CARE**

- C = <u>C</u>heckup. Get complete and regular medical checkups.
- A = <u>A</u>ttention. Pay attention to any new medical symptoms and do not ignore them.
- R = <u>R</u>espect. Respect your body and physical health. They are something special.
- E = <u>E</u>ngage your doctor and partner to achieve best health.

Be *Smart* and actively take *Care* of your physical health every day.

GET A COMPLETE CHECKUP TO UPDATE YOUR SCREENING FOR HEART DISEASE AND CANCER.

Seventy-five percent of the people with heart disease or cancer could be cured today.

Do you believe this? It is true; however, these types of cure rates are not being achieved today because of failure to take advantage of the knowledge and technology that are already available! "Newer and better" need not be the complete focus for good health. With current early detection tests, appropriate therapies, and, most importantly, good lifestyle, most forms of heart disease and cancer can be prevented, cured, stabilized, or even reversed today! The key to improving cure rates is just to enhance your awareness to take advantage of current available medical knowledge and technology while you are still well. So here is what you can do.

Work with your doctor to be sure that your cancer screening is all up to date. This may involve mammograms, colonoscopies, and chest x-rays. You should also check newer technology available, like heart scans and body CT (computed tomography) scans that give excellent pictures of your inside organs. Heart scans can detect early hardening of the arteries, which cause most heart attacks. Body CT scans also detect many early forms of cancer.

These scans have been sometimes criticized for not being necessary or causing harmful radiation. I can say from extensive personal experience that if these scans are done appropriately, neither of the above is true. They are an amazing tool to give you and your doctor very meaningful information about your body. They merely have to be done with consciousness by both you and your physician.

Cancer screening is a big area within medical research. If you have a family history of cancer, discuss this with your doctor as to what type of screening is appropriate for you. Educate yourself. Get appropriate "smart" medical screening tests so that you avoid getting "stupid" preventable diseases.

Here is my list of recommended screening tests. (Make a mental note of areas where you may be deficient for future action plans.)

Basic Recommended Smart Medical Screening Tests to Avoid "Stupid" Illnesses (The Basics)

There really are no "stupid" illnesses, and all illness is not necessarily "preventable." As stated earlier, the value of screening tests is to heighten your awareness earlier in your journey to maintain good health so that you can have earlier corrective action so as to correct or reduce the back-ended effects of illness. It is unlikely that you will need all of the recommended tests below. Work with your doctor in partnership to decide what is best for you.

- Once a year, visit your primary care doctor to review medical care, get a basic laboratory examination, and review any medications you are taking and their potential interactions. Read about potential drug side effects yourself.

- If you are a woman, get basic gynecological care, which includes a pelvic examination, Pap test, and periodic mammogram. Consider breast ultrasound if you have lumpy breasts (fibrocystic disease), a blood test to screen for ovarian cancer, and a vaccination for HPV virus if you are young or have a young daughter who needs vaccination.

- If you are a man, get basic manual prostate examinations with PSA screening blood test. If it is abnormal, consider a prostate ultrasound with possible biopsy. You should examine your testes on a monthly basis for testicular cancer, just the way women need to do a monthly self-breast examination.

- Get a basic screening in the buff of all of your skin for any cancers once per year.

- Update your basic adult immunizations like tetanus, hepatitis B, and pneumo-vax to reduce risk of pneumonia. Ask you doctor if you would benefit from a herpes zoster (shingles) vaccination after age sixty to prevent reactivation of childhood chicken pox.

- Get a complete eye examination of retinas and evaluation for glaucoma once per year.

- Get a periodic hearing evaluation as needed.

- Have regular dental evaluations and get your teeth cleaned at least twice per year. This improves your mouth hygiene, will reduce your risk of heart attack and stroke by decreasing bacteria in the mouth related to these problems, and make you feel better about yourself.

- Have your doctor examine the throat and back of your mouth and neck for potential tumors or swollen lymph nodes.

- Get a manual examination of your thyroid gland to look for lumps. Get a follow-up thyroid scan if abnormal; also, get periodic thyroid function blood tests to see if your thyroid is over- or underactive.

- Get a carotid ultrasound of the neck if you are hypertensive, have elevated cholesterol, are diabetic, or are over seventy to screen for risk of possible stroke.

- Get an abdominal ultrasound to look at your aorta for potential aneurysm and check internal organs for tumors, cysts, or stones.

- Get a screening chest x-ray to evaluate lungs, heart, and aorta. Follow up with a chest CT scan if anything is abnormal.

- Get a baseline screening heart scan at age fifty to evaluate coronary calcification and your risk for heart attack. If abnormal, get a CT coronary angiogram to better evaluate your circulation.

- Have complete blood lipid analysis, particularly if there is any family history of heart disease or if baseline cholesterol is elevated. Also get a baseline homocysteine level, LP(a) test, and CRP level to see if you have an increased risk for heart attack.

- Get an exercise treadmill stress test to evaluate circulation, blood pressure, and heart rhythm. This will help assess your safety for fitness training, particularly after age fifty. If stress test is abnormal, add a heart nuclear scan or echocardiogram of the heart to better evaluate it.

- If you have a heart murmur, enlarged heart, or frequent breathing problems, get a heart echocardiogram to evaluate your heart valves and function of your heart.

- After age fifty, have a baseline abdominal CT scan to screen for cancer.

- Have a colonoscopy at age fifty and every five years to screen for cancer. If you want a non-invasive test, consider a virtual CT colon examination.

- Get a basic bone density examination by DEXA scan or CT scan after age fifty and a periodic follow-up every few years to observe bone loss and potential for bone fractures.

- Get a baseline brain CT examination after age fifty if you are having any neurological complaints (persistent headaches, dizziness, weakness, or change in vision, etc.).

- This list is always incomplete and expanding. Work actively with your primary care doctor to update what is specific for you. Always ask your doctor for better clarification of any of the recommended above tests. Your doctor can often tell you if such tests are covered by your medical insurance. They are more likely to be covered if they are evaluating a medical complaint or symptom. Work with your doctor to navigate the bureaucratic insurance regulations to get your given benefits. You may need to go to a preventive medicine screening clinic to have some of the above tests done. Be prepared that your regular health insurance rarely covers screening tests; however, only you can value your own self-worth. Are you worth spending more than what it takes to fix your car on a regular basis?

Use the benefits of modern medical technology. You are worth it.

The heart CT scan is the best test to see if you have hardening of your heart arteries (atherosclerosis) and are at risk for a heart attack. It is a simple, painless, five-minute test. Check the internet and go to Google ® and type "heart scan" in the search engine. This can help you find a scanning center near you. If you have known heart disease, you will need a more sophisticated heart scan called a cardiac CT coronary angiogram. This is a relatively new test, and it is important to have a physician that is experienced in its interpretation.

The best place that I have seen to get a heart scan is at UCLA Harbor Hospital in Torrance, California. I had the pleasure to train there and work with some of the doctors who pioneered this area of medical research. They are actively involved with research. They do both the simple heart scan to screen for heart disease and the more advanced noninvasive coronary CT angiogram to evaluate people with known heart problems. In fact, I recently had my own heart scanned there to evaluate a recent and, fortunately, minor problem that I had. The center is called the Diagnostic and Wellness Center at UCLA-Harbor. It is located at 1124 West Carson Street, Torrance, California 90502 (phone: 310-222-2772, website: http://www.cardiology. labiomed.org/). Dr. Matthew Budoff is a personal friend. He is the director and an excellent physician, and a world authority in this area of medicine.

If you need a complete medical physical and are willing to travel to Dallas, the Cooper Clinic ® (website: www.cooperaerobics.com) in Dallas, Texas, was founded by Dr. Kenneth Cooper, who is a pioneer in prevention medicine and has over forty years of experience in this area. He wrote the book *Aerobics* in 1968 that changed the way the world exercises today. He and his son Tyler have developed an excellent, coordinated program of baseline evaluation with his gold-standard physical examination, which includes many of the tests listed above. In fact, Dr. Cooper is a friend and helped me review the previous Smart Medical Screening Tests list when I last visited him.

The surroundings at the Cooper Clinic are very pleasant. There is a nice lodge, and a fantastic workout gym and pool are available. Results of tests are reviewed with each client by a physician, usually the same day. The baseline evaluation can be combined with lifestyle programs in nutrition, exercise, and stress management. There are also educational health lectures available.

The above are just two examples from my experience. Research what is available to you locally and what you can afford. There are many excellent local community programs available in preventative health (like YMCA and YWCA) that cost very little. Most community hospitals have regular lectures and programs regarding screening and prevention. Preventative health and education need not be expensive. You need to take advantage of what is nearby, but once again, only you can do the research and have the commitment to get it done.

Questions to Improve Your Physical Health

Journal your responses below

1. What do I already know intuitively that I need to do to improve my health?

2. What medical knowledge do I need to get regarding my own health?

3. What tests do I need to get to update my heart and cancer screening?

4. What bad health habits can I decrease immediately? Do I know the potential side effects of medicines that I am currently taking?

5. How can I partner better with my healthcare providers to improve my health?

6. How can I demonstrate that I truly want to improve my physical health?

7. Am I an exemplar to others in how I take care of my health? What do I need to do to achieve this?

STEP TWO:
IMPROVING YOUR NUTRITIONAL HEALTH

Step Two:

Improving Your Nutritional Health

The next acronym is (FEEL), which will be used to help you remember recommended actions needed to achieve optimal nutrition.

Acronym: **FEEL**
- F = <u>F</u>requently eat foods that promote good health.
- E = <u>E</u>liminate foods that promote illness.
- E = <u>E</u>xperience feeling good by eating healthy foods.
- L = <u>L</u>ove. Make love the secret ingredient of every meal.

To achieve *Optimal* nutrition, think how you ultimately want to *Feel* when you choose what to eat.

RECOMMENDED BASIC IDEAL NUTRITIONAL GOALS:

Food in recent times has been associated with a lot of negativity. This is the last thing you want it to be in your experience. You do not want your life controlled by deprivation, paranoia, and food police. Eating is a very pleasurable experience. You just need to steward that experience with mindful choices.

Most diet programs to lose weight are gimmicks. Most of them work in the short term, and most of them fail in the long term. This is why I stress trying to understand the basics of healthy nutrition and cultivating good food choices that in the long term will make you feel well.

If you eat a healthy diet and combine it with regular exercise, your body will find the size and shape that it was meant to be for the age that you are now.

Since I am often asked what the best diet is, I recommend instead the following general healthy nutritional guidelines as follows:

- Most people need about 2000-3000 calories per day to maintain normal weight and for energy requirements. If you are very active or large-sized, you need more calories. If you are sedentary or small, you need fewer calories. If you want to lose weight, you need to burn more calories than you eat. The bulk of your calories should come from complex carbohydrates and be balanced according to your activity level. Avoid excessive sugar and fat so as not to exceed daily caloric requirements.

- The preferred mix of food is 50 percent complex low-glycemic carbohydrates, 30 percent good-quality protein, and 20 percent good-quality fats, concentrating on unsaturated and monosaturated fats while limiting saturated fats. Increasing omega 3 fatty acids in the diet is highly desirable to reduce risk of heart disease and cancer.

- Eat plenty of fresh organic whole vegetables and fruits daily. Vegetables and fruits are an excellent source of necessary vitamins and minerals. Whole vegetables and fruits contain special properties that prevent heart disease and cancer. Eat a wide variety of these foods that are in season and locally grown. In general, studies have demonstrated that a plant based diet is healthier for you.

- When you eat meat, make it lean. In general, fish and poultry are less fatty than beef. Avoid processed meats. Avoid frying meat and smoked meats. Eat organic meat when possible to avoid hormones, chemicals, and preservatives.

- Enjoy small amounts of alcohol if you like it (one glass of wine or one beer per day). Avoid excesses to limit calories and problems with excessive alcohol.

- Limit salt in your diet. Added salt is rarely needed, since sodium is present in most foods. Daily sodium intake should be limited to no more than 2000-3000 milligrams per day.

- But most importantly, be aware how food affects your body and learn to make adjustments that are specific to your unique genetics and cultural background. Your body changes every ninety days. How you eat today influences what type of body you will have tomorrow. Enjoy good nutrition with friends and family.

Understand Calories: A Calorie is a Calorie is a Calorie and Can Never Be Changed

- A calorie is a measurement of potential energy derived from a food source. It is heat. The higher the calorie content is in food, the higher the potential energy or more heat. Your body is like a furnace. It needs a certain amount of heat in the cells to function. The more you exercise the more calories you need.

- When energy in the form of food is not used, calories are stored. Calories are stored short-term in the liver as glycogen. Calories are stored long-term in the fat cells as fat.

- Complex carbohydrates are your best daily fuel because they are absorbed slowly and metabolized optimally. Complex carbohydrates include food from unrefined grains like whole grain bread, whole grain pasta, brown rice, and yams. Refined carbohydrates like sugar and white bread, regular pasta, and white rice also provide fuel, but are absorbed rapidly into your system. This causes blood glucose (sugar) to rise rapidly and makes metabolizing them less efficient. If you are not doing a lot exercise, this type of glucose absorption is more likely to turn into fat. Calories from fats are very concentrated and should be consumed sparingly.

- The trouble with nutrition today is that we have more calories available than we ever have had in history. This causes wasteful storage and imbalance (a polite way of saying obesity). Counting calories is helpful, but I find it hard to do, and it takes away a lot of the joy of eating.

- A simple evaluation to see if your calories are optimal for what you are doing is whether you feel hot and lethargic or light and energetic.

- Here again, your intuition is the best thermometer. If you have too many calories in your diet, you will feel hot and lethargic. You gain weight easily. If you have the right amount of calories, you will feel energetic and light. However, if you have too few calories, you also will feel cold and lethargic.

You Have to Burn More Calories than You Take In if You Really Want to Lose Weight

One thing that is a truth is that a calorie is a calorie and it can never be changed as a unit. All weight reduction diets are based on this simple truth. There is no other way around this simple truth. When you have an excess of calories, it is called *fat storing*. The reverse is also true that when you take in fewer calories and you burn off more, you will lose weight. This is called *fat burning*. To be fat burning, you need to be active. Turn off your television and go for a walk. This is natural and will restore balance in your life.

Food Diary for a Typical Day of What I Eat

Below is an abbreviated food diary. Choose a typical day to document what you ate and how you felt. Do not make any changes; just maintain your usual pattern of eating. Write down everything you eat and how it is prepared. Include everything you drink. Include each piece of butter, sauce, or condiment.

My Food Diary of a Typical Day (Use either yesterday or today as an example)

Breakfast:

Lunch:

Dinner:

Snacks over 24 Hours:

Was my salt consumption low, medium, or high today?

How much water did I drink today?

Whom did I have meals with, and was I relaxed and enjoying my food and friends?

- Once you have made a diary, then reflect on it. See where you might realistically reduce portions (for example, have one scoop of rice instead of two). Try to give up something that you may not need (for example, soda pop). Or if you decide that you just cannot live without that soda pop, reduce the portion from twenty ounces to ten ounces and from twice a day to once a day. Eat less and eat smaller portions. Become knowledgeable about calorie content, but not obsessive. There are numerous charts and books that list the calorie content of common foods. Read them to become educated about calorie content in food. Read the labels in the stores. (PS: Do not forget to bring your reading glasses with you to the grocery store).

- When you eat at restaurants, ask what sauces are made of and have them on the side. Also, ask to omit extra salting of your food, which acts as a stimulant to appetite. In general, most sauces are very high in calories and salt. Share an entree rather than always having a full entree. Have an appetizer for a meal. Avoid the rich sauces and condiments. Use mustard, which is low in fat and calories, and lemon slices for flavoring.

- Try to avoid or significantly reduce going to fast food restaurants. In general, the food is high in saturated fats, refined carbohydrates, and salt. Because food is stored for long periods of time, trans-fats and preservatives are common at these restaurants or in any foods that are stored on the grocery shelves for months. The healthiest strategy is just to avoid them.

- Know the food you eat and its approximate calorie content. Estimate your need for calories by how much exercise you have done or are going to do. If you do this, you will eat more the way you *need* to eat, rather than the way you *want* to eat.

- Make simple changes and adjustments over time. Over time, these simple changes will pay big dividends.

To keep weight optimal, it is desirable to have bulky, low dense calorie food.

- One of the most useful concepts that I have observed is relationship between calorie density and bulk of food. The concept goes like this: most people will eat about two to three pounds of food per day to get a full sensation and relieve hunger. Foods that are bulky yet low in calories, like vegetables and steamed potatoes, are more desirable than food that are small and high in dense calories, like cheese or sauces.

- Food density changes when it is processed. As an example, a baked potato with mustard is high in bulk and relatively low in calories. However, as a potato is fried and absorbs oil and is turned into a French fry and then is dipped in a sweet sauce, the potato loses its bulk and becomes dense in calories. As it becomes a potato chip, special oils (trans-fats) are added to preserve its shelf life. Choose to make your food choices more natural and "live," and you will be healthier.

- Another example is eating a whole orange compared to drinking orange juice. A single orange is low in calories and high in fiber. It takes a while to peel one orange and eat it. However, orange juice is derived from many oranges and has decreased fiber. It becomes high in dense or concentrated calories. The problem worsens if corn syrup (high fructose sugar) is added to increase sweetness. Soda drinks are the worst offenders, as they are almost pure high fructose corn syrup. Wine and beer are also concentrated calories. If you are consuming a lot of the above beverages, you may find it very difficult to lose weight. Do not forget that water has no calories. Do not be afraid to ask just for water (even at a fast food restaurant or a bar).

- Foods likes butter are very high dense calorie foods and should definitely be limited if you want to lose weight. Be aware of how much butter is used in restaurant cooking and in desserts. Sometimes, it is helpful just to read a recipe book of fine dining just to see how much butter and sugar are in food so as to restrict or avoid those things when tempted.

By eating bulky but low dense calorie foods, you can actually eat more and weigh less. This is the basis of the so-called "Hawaiian diet." This diet gets back to the way Hawaiians ate in the past. It includes high amounts of plant-based foods that are simply prepared without sauces and small amounts of protein from seafood or lean meats.

I have seen people lose significant amounts of weight by returning to this "old" diet, particularly when combined with regular aerobic exercise. They are definitely healthier. Their diabetes, high blood pressure, and cholesterol levels all improve when they have this bulky diet combined with exercise. People generally enjoy this type of diet because it fills them up.

MOST IMPORTANTLY: PREPARE MOST OF YOUR OWN FOOD

Preparing more of your own food is critical to taking charge of improving your own nutrition. This is what people have always done until recent times. Restaurants are convenient, delicious, and fun, but there is nothing healthier than home cooking. Below are some samples of simple recipes that I developed as examples to help you improve your food choices and nutrition.

Three Simple, Healthy Meals (If I Can Make These Meals, Anyone Can)

Breakfast:

Try **oatmeal** (good for you and fills you up).

- Buy old-fashioned oatmeal from a store that sells in bulk or bins. Avoid processed, packaged oatmeal with additives, as it is high in salt and sugar.

- Before bedtime, get a large bowl. Add desired amount of oatmeal to bowl. Add enough water to soak oats overnight (usually about 1 cup per serving), Heat in microwave for one minute and let it stand there overnight.

- In morning, oatmeal is ready to eat. You can eat it either cold (it will have more fiber and be less glycemic) or hot. Just add a little more water if it is dry. Heat in microwave for one to two minutes if you want it hot. Let it cool and eat.

- Add condiments such as fresh papayas, bananas, berries, walnuts, ground whole flax seeds, cinnamon (good to lower blood pressure), and low-fat milk (or soy, rice, or almond milk). Add a small amount of honey for sweetness as desired.

- Eat and enjoy with a good dark roast coffee or tea. (Use decaf if you are sensitive to caffeine.)

This simple meal can be varied every day with available fruit and nuts. It is fast, cheap, and easy to make. It will give you energy in the morning and decrease cravings for sweets. It helps to lower bad LDL cholesterol. It gives you fiber for good bowel movement. The fruit with ground flax seeds gives you vitamins, fiber, and omega 3 fatty acids in your diet.

Lunch:

Brown Rice and Beans with Vegetables (good and saves you money when you avoid fast food restaurants).

- Buy organic brown rice, dried red beans, and whole flax seeds.

- Cook rice and beans together in a rice cooker (use about 1 cup of rice, ⅓ cup beans, and 1 tablespoon flax seeds). Have a little extra water compared to when making white rice and cook a little longer.

- After cooking, you can add cut-up parts of ginger root and walnuts and season with Braggs Aminos® (soy sauce substitute).

- Keep in refrigerator overnight to store.

- When getting ready to go to work in morning or when wanting to make a quick lunch, take one scoop of rice and beans and put in microwavable glass container. On top, add cut vegetables like broccoli, bok choy, zucchini, or whatever is desired or in season. Add a few walnuts or almonds as condiments for taste.

- Bring to work. At lunchtime, either eat cold or reheat in microwave briefly and eat warm.

- Drink with plenty of water flavored with a lemon slice for flavor.

The rice and beans is a base and can be kept for days in the refrigerator. Keep plenty of fresh vegetables and nuts as additives and experiment with different combinations.

Another quick and easy lunch:

Steamed Sweet Potatoes, Yams, or Pumpkin Squash with Sauces (very easy to make and store in refrigerator for when needed)

- Buy organic sweet potatoes, yams, or different kinds of squash.

- Either the night before work or in the morning, cut slices of potatoes or squash. Steam cook for about 20 minutes until soft. Remove. Put in a glass container.

- On top of potatoes, add for taste either honey (for sweet taste), chili hot sauce (for spicy taste), or small amounts of Braggs Aminos ® (a relatively low-salt soy sauce alternative). Take to work and eat either hot (reheat in microwave for 1 minute) or cold.

Both of the above lunches are easy, cheap, and healthier than any fast food alternative that you will buy. Pack your lunch and eat it with friends in the park. This will make your lunch more soulful. You will save a lot of money and have more energy. You can vary the above recipes with multiple condiments and experiment with your own variations. By making your own lunch, you take control of what goes in your body.

Dinner:

Lightly Stir-fried Noodles and Shrimp with Vegetables (easy to make and will impress your friends).

- Buy shrimp, desired vegetables, ginger root, garlic, and fresh, homemade rice noodles.

- Have a large stir-fry style pan with lid. Cut up garlic and ginger to desired taste. I recommend using plenty of garlic and ginger if you like the taste. Set aside in dish.

- Buy fresh, whole shrimp with shells still on. Wash and set aside.

- Cut vegetables (whatever desired: broccoli, eggplant, okra, bok choy, onions, all with short cooking times). You can add a splash of Braggs ® apple cider vinegar to vegetables to bring out taste.

- When using fresh noodles, cooking time is only about 2 minutes. (If using dried noodles, you will need to cook these ahead of time and then set aside in large bowl). Set aside in large bowl.

- In pan, add small amount of olive oil to bottom of pan. Cook on relatively low to medium heat and add garlic and ginger. Add shrimp. Stir and cook for about 3-5 minutes, until shells of shrimp turn red.

- Add vegetables and noodles. Add just a little water to create steam. Put lid on pan and cook for 1-2 minutes.

- Watch heat carefully and turn off heat quickly so as to not overcook. Remove from pan and garnish with fresh Chinese parsley.

- Serve and eat immediately with a glass of favorite wine or a bottle of cold spring water.

You can prepare the above meal before your guests arrive. When your guests arrive, have a glass of wine and chat. When ready for dinner, just heat your pan and prepare this meal in minutes in front of them. When they taste it, I am sure that they will ask for seconds.

The above dinner can be varied by substituting pieces of fresh fish, clams, mussels, chicken, or tofu. You can add different condiments, like fresh basil or mint, depending on taste. Experiment and enjoy the journey!

Remember the most important thing with any meal that you prepare or enjoy: the secret ingredient for success and good health is love.

There is a wise saying below that I have embellished:

"Better a meal of vegetables with love than the fattened calf with hatred" (Adapted from Proverbs 15:17). Have that meal in a loving setting with friends and family, and it is even better.

If you make healthy choices as described above and combine this with regular exercise, you will begin to feel better in three weeks. Remain patient and focus on the long-term goal of being healthy rather than a quick fix of being thin.

QUESTIONS TO IMPROVE YOUR NUTRITIONAL HEALTH

Journal your action plans below.

1. I know that I can feel better if I eat better and make some changes as follows:

2. I need to educate myself more on basic nutrition in the following way:

3. These are the foods that I want to increase in my diet:

4. These are foods that I want to limit that I know that I have in excess:

5. These are foods that I want to try to totally eliminate from my diet that I know are potentially harmful to my health:

6. This is how I want to express my gratefulness for the food:

7. This is how I want to eat more with friends and family:

STEP THREE:
IMPROVING YOUR FITNESS HEALTH

STEP THREE:

IMPROVING YOUR FITNESS AND INTERACTION WITH OTHERS

The third acronym is (DO), to help you remember areas to improve both your physical and expressive motion in life.

Acronym: **DO**

- **D** = **D**aily. Focus each day on doing something both physical and expressive.
- **O** = **O**ptimal. Find and adjust to what is optimal for you.

To achieve *Age Appropriate* motion, ask yourself every day what you really want to *Do* physically and expressively with your life.

Understanding How Oxygen works with the Body and Its Relationship to Activity

- Oxygen utilization by the body is closely correlated with your endurance. This is called aerobic utilization. Oxygen and fuel are both needed for muscles to work properly. Good nutrition provides your fuel.

- A measure of ability to utilize oxygen is called VO2Max. The better your body utilizes oxygen, the higher your VO2Max will be. The higher your VO2Max is, the more endurance you will have.

- Measuring VO2Max is rarely done during routine checkups. Generally, it is a research technique. Professional athletes may get a VO2Max determination as part of an evaluation for a training program.

- VO2Max is measured during an exercise treadmill stress test. A claustrophobic mask is fitted over your face during exercise to measure exhaled gases. The test is much more involved than a standard treadmill stress test. When you are finished with the test, gases that you exhaled are measured and VO2Max is determined. The higher your VO2Max, the more fit you are aerobically.

- VO2Max is in part determined by heredity, like muscle fiber composition. But just like muscle composition, its maximum potential is reached only with regular exercise. As VO2Max goes up, you feel better and stronger. You breathe better with exercise. If you are starting with a low VO2Max, regular aerobic exercise will make you feel much stronger in just three weeks. This is the positive effect of training.

- VO2Max does not stay the same for very long. Another way of stating this is that you cannot store exercise. It has a short memory. This gets worse as you age. It takes you longer to get into shape, and it goes away faster than when you were young. VO2Max is changing every day depending on your activity level. The higher your activity level is on a regular basis, the higher your VO2Max will be.

- You always have a potentially high unused capacity to increase VO2Max. This reserve decreases with age but never goes away. VO2Max can still be improved markedly at any age. This is why many older people who are retired and exercise regularly actually have better endurance than when they were younger and not exercising. There is no need to slow down as you age. In fact, as you age, regular activity is even more important to maintain health and fitness. Once again, "To rest is to rust"!

- Oxygen comes from the air you breathe and is influenced by elevation. If you go up to a very high mountain, the level of oxygen drops in the environment and you feel it. (Also, most airplane travel is equivalent to being on a 10,000 foot mountain, as the oxygen level is reduced in the cabin unless extra oxygen is added.) When on top of a tall mountain, you breathe harder to make up for lack of oxygen. It is harder to exercise at high altitude. If your VO2Max is high, you are less likely to feel the effects of higher elevation.

- Sometimes, the body benefits from higher-than-normal oxygen levels. This is done by breathing from a concentrated oxygen tank. Oxygen is used to treat people with heart attacks and strokes to try to preserve tissue when it has been stressed. High-dose oxygen treatment is used to treat scuba diving injuries and also used for very high mountain climbing.

Fuel for Exercise and Calories

- In addition to oxygen, the muscles need a steady supply of glucose (sugar) to contract. This is your main source of fuel. You get a continuous source of glucose in your blood from the food you eat.

- Once again, the short-term fuel is stored as glycogen in the liver and in the long-term, it is stored as fat. The body has a complex metabolism that changes glucose, glycogen, and fat continuously, depending upon your energy requirements.

- Fat is a richer fuel than glucose or glycogen. It takes more exercise to burn a molecule of fat than it does a molecule of glucose. That is why it is the most difficult to burn off body fat.

- When you burn a molecule of glucose, it releases a specific calorie of energy. This is how calories and glucose are related. The more you exercise, the more calories you burn. The less you exercise, the fewer calories you burn. When you have excess fuel that is not burned, it is stored for a later use.

- One pound of body fat has the capacity to burn 3500 calories. Fat is very important for survival as an emergency reserve for energy metabolism. However, the problem today for many of us is that we have more fat reserves than what we need. Food is readily available, and we do not have famines. Body fat builds up insidiously and also disappears slowly. Body fat only goes away with sustained, regular exercise.

- When you exercise, the first source of fuel that you utilize is glucose. Glycogen from the liver is mobilized when glucose in the blood starts to become depleted. The last source of fuel to be used is fat. It is important to understand this relationship if you want to lose fat. For the first twenty minutes of aerobic exercise, glucose is the predominant source of fuel. It is only after twenty minutes of steady exercise that body fat starts to be mobilized and burns. This is why increasing the duration of exercise is important if you want to lose body fat.

- Weightlifting improves how your muscles utilize glucose. It increases your metabolism so that glucose that you eat is burned more efficiently. Combining lifting small weights with aerobic exercise is a good strategy to increase your baseline metabolism.

- A sustained negative calorie balance is needed to burn sufficient fat reserves to lose weight. As an example, with simple walking, about 400 calories are burned per hour. Therefore, to burn off one pound of fat, it would take almost nine hours of sustained walking. More vigorous exercise will burn more calories faster; however, this comes mostly from calories derived from glucose, and when this gets low, you stop exercising because of fatigue before you start to burn fat.

- In a weight reduction program, your goal should be to lose about one pound per week. When you lose more weight rapidly, this is mostly weight from fluid rather than fat and is prone to return quickly when you stop dieting.

The simple and unavoidable truth is that if your goal is to lose fat, you must remember that a program of sustained exercise over months combined with reduced calorie intake is the only sure way to lose weight.

It is best to make little daily changes in your diet and exercise program which are sustainable habits, rather than big, sudden changes that cause too much pain and are not sustainable. Omit that once-a-day café latte and muffin. Do not use butter on your bread. Do not have a soda drink when you are thirsty or out of habit. Walk the stairs. Get out of your car and walk whenever you can. Walk to the gym. Walk to a restaurant. These are the little changes that will all add up over a year to a negative calorie balance and weight reduction.

MINIMUM EXERCISE RECOMMENDATIONS

You need a minimum of forty-five minutes of aerobic exercise four times per week for your health to be optimal. This will make you feel physically better within three weeks. To increase your VO2Max (measurement of your body's ability to utilize oxygen), you will need more intense exercise. Below are of examples of typical calories burned with different activities.

Walking is the most natural and common way to achieve regular daily aerobic motion. Walking has a significant advantage because it is weight-bearing (carrying the weight of the body). Weight-bearing exercise tends to strengthen both muscles and bones. Walking can also be done indoors on a treadmill. A treadmill is helpful for doing exact measurements of speed and calorie consumption. A treadmill is also helpful if it is too hot or too cold outside and it is raining. Jogging or running is more intense than walking. These activities burn more calories and increase VO2Max to higher levels; however, duration is more important for good health than intensity. A short run may have less benefit than a long walk.

- Slow walking (3 miles per hour) burns 300 calories/hour.
- Brisk walking (4 miles per hour) burns 400 calories/hour.
- Slow jogging (5 miles per hour) burns 500 calories per hour.
- Faster jogging (6 miles per hour) burns 650 calories per hour.
- Fast running (7 miles per hour) burns 800 calories per hour.

It is easier and more efficient for most people to increase duration rather than intensity. Intense running is hard for most people to sustain over time and is also hard on the muscles and joints. Therefore, using shorter bursts of running can be helpful as interval training when combined with walking. Changing pace from walking to jogging in cycles will maintain endurance and gradually build up VO2Max. This will burn more calories.

Hiking is an extension of walking. It has the advantage of seeing nature and experiencing the outdoors. Since it is usually done over hours, it is sustained exercise and good at improving VO2Max and burning fat.

- Mild-level hiking burns about 400 calories per hour.
- Moderate hiking up and down hills burns about 600 calories per hour.
- Intense hiking up hills burns about 800-900 calories per hour.

- High altitude hiking burns 1000 calories per hour.

The elliptical cross trainer machine is a specialized exercise machine that simulates walking and arm movement. Tension can be adjusted to make the exercise more difficult. It is good at burning calories and improving VO2Max while at the same time being easier on the joints than running. Other machines, such as stair climbers and rowing machines, are also very helpful in increasing VO2Max and burning calories.

- Low-level elliptical training burns 400 calories per hour.
- Moderate elliptical training burns 600 calories per hour.
- Intense elliptical training burns 800 calories per hour.

Bicycling is an excellent alternative or supplement to a regular walking program. Bicycling uses different muscles and can be easier on the joints. Outdoor bicycling is a way to enjoy fresh air and gets you from one place to another efficiently. If you can use it as a regular mode of transportation, this is not only good for you, but additionally, you will save money on your gasoline bills.

Stationary bicycling is an excellent alternative for indoor regular cycling. This can be combined with reading or watching television or listening to music to enhance the experience. Intense bicycling can be done in the form of a spinning class which includes intense interval training.

- Mild bicycling (8 miles per hour) burns 300 calories per hour.
- Moderate bicycling (10-12 miles per hour) burns 450 calories per hour.
- Intense bicycling burns 600-800 calories per hour.

Swimming is an excellent way to maintain aerobic fitness and muscle tone and is easy on the joints. Regular swimming has been demonstrated to increase longevity. Freshwater swimming or pool swimming is harder to do because the body is less buoyant and the work of staying afloat is harder. In the ocean, you are more buoyant, meaning you float easier. This makes ocean swimming easier. However, swimming against the current makes the exercise more difficult and builds greater VO2Max.

Swimming can be taught at all ages, and even non-swimmers can participate in water aerobic exercises in a pool. Swimming with a mask and fins can enhance swimming and make it easier. Using fins will exercise different leg and back muscles.

- Water aerobics burns about 400-500 calories per hour.
- Moderate lap swimming burns about 500-700 calories per hour.
- Vigorous lap swimming burns 800-900 calories per hour.

Different sports can be very aerobic and enjoyable and social at the same time. In general, sports that involve more sustained running, like soccer and basketball, build greater VO2Max. However, any sport is helpful, and the most important component is that it is enjoyable. It is better to participate in sports rather than be a spectator, where there is no improvement in aerobic capacity. Examples of calories burned in sports are as below.

- Soccer: 800 calories per hour
- Basketball: 750 calories per hour
- Singles tennis: 500-600 calories per hour
- Doubles tennis 400-500 calories per hour
- Downhill skiing: 400-700 calories per hour
- Cross-country skiing: 500-900 calories per hour
- Roller skating: 400-500 calories per hour
- Judo class: 300-600 calories per hour
- Boxing class: 400-800 calories per hour
- Golf with walking: 400-500 calories per hour
- Golf with cart: 200 calories per hour
- Bowling: 200-300 calories per hour
- Watching sports on television: 25 calories per hour!

Daily activities can also be aerobic and enjoyable while accomplishing tasks. Here are a few examples of work-related activities that can be aerobic.

- Cleaning house: 300-400 calories per hour
- Washing the car: 300-400 calories per hour
- Walking the dog: 300-400 calories per hour
- Gardening: 300-400 calories per hour
- Digging with a shovel: 500-800 calories per hour
- Moving rocks: 500-800 calories per hour
- Shoveling snow: 600-800 calories per hour

Enjoyable activities that burn calories:

- Ballroom dancing: 300 calories per hour
- Aerobic dancing: 400-500 calories per hour
- Intimate activity with a loved one: 200-300 calories per hour!

Do not obsess trying to remember calorie levels associated with different activities.

Just remember your intensity and duration and how you feel. Try to do a number of different things so that you cross-train and use different muscles. As you age, try to exercise whatever is not hurting that day!

- With all aerobic activity, it is good to have a warm-up period of low-level exercise and a cooling down phase at the end of exercise. The body responds better to gradual change in metabolism rather than abrupt changes.

- Stretching before and after exercise is important for optimal muscle function and flexibility. This also prevents muscle injury.

- Interval training is very helpful to increase your VO2Max. Interval training alternates different levels of low, moderate, and strenuous activity. It can be adjusted to almost any aerobic activity, like walking, running, bicycling, or other activities. By having periods of intense exercise, this stresses the body in a good way to increase the VO2Max over time and improve endurance. It also tends to strengthen the muscles.

- Mixing walking with running is a good way to cover long distances. This is what our ancestors did when they hunted for food. You can run a marathon this way. You can jog for ten minutes and then walk for five minutes. You repeat this timing until the marathon is finished. This allows your muscles to recover and prevents lactic acid from building up in the muscles. It also prevents overuse.

Helpful Ideas to Improve Fitness:

As you develop you own action plans in this area, here are a few practical suggestions that you might want to consider.

- Buy a pedometer. A pedometer measures the number of steps that you take over a period of time. Research has demonstrated that if you measure your steps from the moment you wake up to the moment you go to sleep at night, you should take at least 10,000 steps per day for optimal health. This may sound like a lot of steps; however, every little bit of motion adds up in a full day. Most people in the past easily took 10,000 steps per day when they did not have cars or other conveniences. Today, the average person takes only about 2,000-3,000 steps per day. This is far less than what the body needs to maintain optimal health. If you swim or bicycle for thirty minutes, add 5,000 steps to your total. If you use an elliptical trainer, add 5,000 steps for thirty minutes that you use the machine.

- Buy a small, fold-up bicycle and use it. I did it. I ride my little bicycle all over downtown Honolulu. I get to places faster than most cars during heavy traffic. I save money on gasoline. I meet new friends. I enjoy the fresh air and scenery. I feel healthier and empowered being able to provide my own energy for transportation. These bicycles have become widely available. They are easy to ride and a great way to get around for short journeys that you would otherwise drive in the car to reach. When you go shopping, to the movies, to a restaurant, to work, or to the gym, think of using a cycle rather than a car.

- Buy some small weights to do arm exercises. You can store these under your bed and exercise while you are watching television. This is a great way to add definition to your body mass, and it improves your metabolism of sugar.

- Get bold—do something out of your comfort zone. Take a hike in nature. Play a physical game with your kids rather than watch television.

- Balance your exercise with stretching and yoga. Do not ignore recovery. Get a relaxing massage, take a sauna, or have a glass of wine with a friend in a Jacuzzi. Enjoy life.

QUESTIONS TO IMPROVE YOUR FITNESS AND INTERACTION WITH PEOPLE

Journal your responses below:

1. When I stand naked in front of the mirror, what do I see? Is that the reflection that I want it to be?

2. What are the basics of physical fitness that I need to know more about?

3. What aerobic exercise do I need to increase?

4. What type of strength training and flexibility training do I need to do?

5. How can I sleep better? Is there something that I am not dealing with? What are other things I need to do to nurture my body and rejuvenate?

6. How can I specifically better balance giving with receiving?

7. What do I really want to *do* with my life?

Introduction to Improving Your Spiritual Health:

Improving your body physically with a proper medical checkup, good nutrition, and good exercise will build your physical confidence. This will then allow you to address your most important area of health, which is spiritual health.

The last but most important area to address with this workbook is improving the quality of all of your relationships.

This is a morning prayer that I learned from a Sherpa while climbing a mountain together in Tibet. It is a very old Sanskrit prayer that I will translate into modern English as follows:

Today, I will grow older.
Someday, I will get sick.
Someday, I will die.
I will lose everything I have, including possessions, physical health, and friends and family.
What only remains are my actions.
So as I start this day, let my actions to be positive and help me to look for opportunities where I can serve others.

STEP FOUR:
IMPROVING YOUR SPIRITUAL HEALTH

STEP FOUR:

IMPROVING YOUR SPIRITUAL HEALTH

Your spiritual health is the most important component of your health and, in the long term, will ultimately determine sickness or wellness. It is also the area where you potentially have the greatest direction and control in your life. Unfortunately, it is also the most neglected.

Here is the last acronym (BE), to introduce this section.

Acronym: **BE**

- B = Believe that anything is possible.
- E = Experience this wonderful life through relationships. That is why you are here.

To achieve *Rich Relationships*, focus every day on who you really want to *Be* and make it happen with your actions.

WHAT ARE RICH RELATIONSHIPS?

- Relationships with yourself, others, your ancestors, and a higher spirit are all synchronous and continuous. However, all relationships begin with you and how you feel about yourself. You get back what you give out.

- The most important question regarding the status of your spiritual health is "Do you feel worthy?" Everyone will have periods during his or her life when self-worth is challenged. The paradox to overcoming difficulties with self-worth is not to continually reflect on unworthiness or being a victim, but to use adversity to build character. If you feel negatively about yourself, you need to change your attitude. You have the ability to do this every second of the day. Do not replay constant negativity in your brain.

- When you are feeling depressed or anxious, make a conscious choice to replace negative thoughts with positive thoughts. Put yourself in a positive environment. This will lead to positive actions. When stuck in the rut of unworthiness, the best way to change the situation is to find ways to serve others. When you do this, you will make heart-to-heart connections that will strengthen you and improve your self-worth. This, in turn, will build your own character, which will be lasting. "Treat others as you would like to be treated" is one of the best and oldest universal pieces of self-help advice.

- Another area that affects everyone is trans-generational behaviors. These are behaviors and emotions that have been handed down to you from your parents or surrogate parents and even distant ancestors that you do not know. Trans-generational behaviors, particularly traumas and stresses, may go back several generations. They cause you to have unexpected anxieties and depression without knowing where they come from. These behaviors often lead to abusive behavior, drug addiction, and/or alcoholism.

- You have the power to change the cycle and modify any trans-generational behaviors so as to improve your own health and so as not to transmit negative behaviors to your children. Try to become aware of these unexpected behaviors that are inside of you. Become aware without blaming anyone. This is the first step in changing negative trans-generational behaviors. Once again, use adversity from inherited behaviors to build character, rather than becoming a victim of circumstances.

- Everyone is going to have periods when he/she feels anxious in his/her spiritual heart. This is the very time that your heart needs a message of reassurance. This support can come from within, someone else, or a higher spirit. This is the real value of *all* relationships. Ultimately, to get encouragement when you need it, you have to cultivate your relationships and keep your own heart open to comfort others.

- Improving relationships is the most important thing that you can do to improve both your physical and spiritual health. Unfortunately, this area of your health is often most neglected. You tend to take relationships for granted. You think good relationships will just happen and that broken relationships will just heal. Neither is true. Rather than committing to positive improvement in your relationships, you often drift with the wind. When your relationships drift, you fail to achieve your full potential and lose your destiny. You will also keep repeating relational problems; however, this is an area where you potentially have great choice and control to determine the quality of your life.

- Regardless of faith or religion, I have never met a person who has never felt a higher spirit working at some point in his or her life. Following a particular faith or religion is a personal choice. I do know, however, that you have to make time to connect and appreciate all of the miracles of the universe around you each day. This is the most important part in breaking one's own trance to become connected to a greater energy within the universe. Everyone will find his or her own particular path in doing this. I personally recommend spending time enjoying the beauties of nature to get you to realize that life is greater than yourself.

- Spirituality is vague and different for everyone. It is often connected with religious teachings. To avoid religious conflict, I recommend the secular approach of improving your spirituality by focusing on improving your relationships with yourself, others, and a higher spirit; however, you interpret that to be. All of these relationships act simultaneously in your life, whether you want it or not. Through your actions, you will determine the quality of these relationships.

Love Yourself and You Will Connect with the Universal Love

Love is really a continuum. Love of self, others, and a higher spirit are all one. There is room in life to respect all religions. Tolerance is very important. We are all different and may see the same truths a little differently, depending on where we are in our own personal evolution.

How do you improve relationships with a higher spirit? Merely love and be loved. This is what your spiritual heart really wants.

Here are a few practical hints for a better relationship with a higher spirit and to feel a higher spirit working in your life. These recommendations are universal and nondenominational.

- Put yourself in a position to experience the wonder and beauty of this universe. Nature is beautiful and perfect. It is also a great teacher.

- Realize that you are surrounded by nature wherever you are. Whether it is beautiful or ugly just depends on your perspective. Appreciate it for whatever it is and appreciate it now.

- Develop a spirit of gratefulness. Let your heart be grateful for everything because everything is perfect every day. Realize that gifts of health, food, and relationships come from beyond you. Everything is interconnected. When things do not seem to go right, remember this lesson.

- Be aware that your living today is the result of billions of years before you. Feel this in every cell of your body. You are here for a reason.

- Remember how many times your life has been threatened and you were not harmed. Why do you think this is so?

- Be humble. You are not the center of the universe. Humility builds relationships. Pride destroys relationships. This is true for developing a relationship with a higher spirit.

- Give forgiveness freely. Do not hold onto it and ration it. When you forgive, it is your heart that heals. You are better. Be active to forgive quickly and spread grace freely. Forgiveness does not condone wrong actions by someone else. It simply removes your judgmental mind, which can become compulsive and destructive. Being unforgiving not only causes stress on you; it robs you of the future by being constantly tied to the past.

- Hope is what sustains your actions. Take away hope and you have taken away a man's life. Maintaining hope of optimal health and life is a sustaining force in moving you in the right direction. True faith is being sure of what you hope for and certain of what you cannot see.

- Most importantly, let your actions be guided by a loving heart. It is easy for your actions to be self-serving. But ultimately, your heart grows richer if you serve more than you receive. This is another fundamental spiritual truth, that if you love, you will be loved.

All of the above things are already in your heart and will connect you closer to a higher spirit, whatever your faith. You just need to access them. When your heart is balanced, you will naturally practice these habits. When you are aware, you will know quickly when you are out of balance and self-correct. As you do these actions, you will experience awe in your heart, which will connect you to a relationship with a higher spirit.

Exercises to Improve Your Spiritual Fitness:

Just like you need physical exercise to improve your physical fitness, you need spiritual exercises to improve your relationships if you want them to be rich. Below are some spiritual exercises designed to improve your relationships with yourself, others, and a higher spirit. They start off relatively easy and become progressively more challenging.

Exercise #1: Change your attitude in a nanosecond with a smile.

Remember:

"An anxious heart weighs a man down, but a kind word cheers him up" (adapted from Proverbs 12:25).

Make an effort to smile more over the next week. Try to smile at five people that you would not have ordinarily smiled at each day, like people on an elevator, or on a bus, or at work, or in the park. Give them a pleasant "Hello." Keep a mental record of these events and see how it changes both your interaction and, more importantly, how you even feel about yourself. See how what you give out will come back to you. Smile particularly at people that seemed stressed or worried and see if you can improve their attitude. It is contagious. Waking up begins with the right attitude.

Exercise #2: Everyone has a story. Enrich your life by learning about others' stories.

Over the next five days, find one person each day and actively listen and find out about his or her life. See how this changes your own life and your interaction with that person. Find a way to tell your own story, be it in writing, painting, music, or dance. Everyone has a story to tell, and we are all enriched by hearing others' stories.

EXERCISE #3: OVERCOME THE MONKEY MIND.

This story was told to me many years ago by a guru at an ashram in southern India:

There is a story in ancient India as to how to catch a monkey by appealing to his desires or wants. In southern India, they have big clay pots that have narrow tops and big bases. They are quite heavy. Monkeys find these pots amusing. To catch a monkey, you get a sweet and put it in the bottom of the pot. The monkey comes by at night when no one is watching and smells the sweet and reaches into the big pot to get it. However, with a clenched fist holding the sweet, the monkey cannot get his hand out of the pot. The pot is too heavy to move. The monkey panics and just keeps trying harder and harder to get the clenched fist out of the pot, but cannot do it. In the morning, the monkey is worn out and lying next to the pot with his hand still in the pot. All the monkey had to do to regain his freedom was to let go of the sweet or desire. By holding on, he has lost his freedom.

This holding on to desires at the expense of your freedom is called the *monkey mind*. It is important to overcome the monkey mind to be free and healthy. The monkey mind is still with us today. We are no different from a monkey. We are all tempted by sweet desires. One of our biggest sweets today is use of credit cards.

If you have a monkey mind, it is easy to make getting money your top priority in life. Money is very sweet. I have seen this cause more stress and illness as a physician than any other thing. The pursuit of accumulation of money and spending and buying things can easily become a priority in our commercial society. Advertising fuels this adverse appetite and imbalance. You start to think that you actually need all of those things that you are bombarded with daily in advertisements. But the dark side is debt and stress. I have had patients with totally normal hearts get heart attacks over stresses related to money.

If you do not have money, you often feel that you are a failure. You feel unworthy. Nothing could be less true. Remember always, "You were born worthy, and only you can make yourself feel unworthy." Only you can make yourself feel deprived. Only you can make yourself stressed by debt and make it the focus of your thinking. You do need to be responsible with stewarding money well, but "What you think about, you become." It is true that the best things in life are free. Deprivation can in most cases be an asset and enhance health. Good relationships do not come through money. They come through time.

A sense of achievement and relaxation do not come through money. Money, like anything, should be managed well, with discipline, but it should not be your "god" or ruling force. It is you worship money; you will quickly be out of balance, because money is a "false god." To maintain balance, look at your priorities: what you think may be deprivation may be your biggest asset. Spending time with your family at the beach or in the mountains is free. Pursuit of money can distract you from your family, which is one of your most important relationships.

On your deathbed, your kids will remember the time you spent with them, not the money you give them. It is all a matter of perception as to what is important and having the right perception can lead to good health. You just have to let go of the sweet.

Write below what you are holding on to that is limiting your freedom. Are you willing to let go of it?

EXERCISE #4: FOCUS ON THE PRESENT MOMENT.

I was once told the secret of depression and anxiety in a very simple way. It is as follows:

If you think too much about the past, you will be depressed.
If you think too much about the future, you will be anxious.
Focus on the present moment and you will be content.

The past, present, and future are a continuum. Appreciate this.

Write below things that you think too much about in the past:

Write below things that you think too much about the future:

Think about how your actions in the present can influence your perception of the past and prepare you for the future.

Now are you ready for more difficult realizations? If so, proceed.

Exercise #5: All rich relationships begin with you.

All relationships always start with you. How you feel about your worth is the most important thing in how you will feel towards others and their worth. Once you realize this, it will make you understand all of your relationships better. If your relationships are not what you want them to be, look at yourself first. Regain your self-worth. Paradoxically, this often happens through service to others.

Think of ways in which you would like to serve others and write this down below:

Exercise #6: All rich relationships are heart-to-heart connections.

Your have a connection between you and your spiritual heart. You also have a connection to other people's spiritual hearts and to a higher spirit. The universal spiritual heart is omnipresent and connects us all. These connections make up your relationships. The more you positively access these connections, the richer and healthier your life will be.

Write down below the names of people with whom you would like to have closer heart-to-heart connections:

Exercise #7: Everyone is worthy, and of equal merit.

The only one who can take away your self-worth is you. Self-worth is the single most important thing for good spiritual and physical health. If you have lost your self-worth, you particularly need to connect to your spiritual heart.

If this is hard for you, this is a particularly crucial time to try to connect heart to heart with someone else and, even more importantly connect, to the energy of the universal omnipresent spiritual heart. Self-worth cannot be taught in a classroom or be learned from a book. It just needs to be experienced. However, if someone is abusing you, it is your responsibility to avoid that person.

Without self-worth, you will never thrive. Self-worth costs nothing. It is just recognizing a gift you already have. But you can lose this gift. The good news is that you can begin to restore a broken relationship with your spiritual heart through awareness.

Is there someone you need to avoid that is abusing you? Write it down and how you are going to avoid them. In what ways are you going to build up your self-worth?

Exercise #8: It is possible to mend broken relationships.

This takes work and commitment from both parties to be effective. It will not happen on its own. At some point, everyone's relationship with his or her spiritual heart will be stressed by life events and interactions with other people. This is a time when you particularly need to connect with your spiritual heart or consciousness for direction.

This will be one of your greatest challenges of your life. Broken relationships can be with self, others, or a higher spirit and are always interconnected. Broken relationships, more than anything, contribute to low esteem. All of these relationships are repairable. When you work to repair these relationships, you will be stronger and healthier.

What broken relationships do you need to work on? Write them below and ask your spiritual heart for direction.

Exercise #9: What do you want your legacy to be? Realize the importance of living your legacy now.

Your greatest legacy will always be your relationships. Relationships are with yourself, others, and a higher spirit and are always interconnected. You feel worthy through all of your relationships. As a cardiologist, I have been at the bedside at the time of death of many of my patients. When people are near death, they are very focused on what is important in life. They do not want to be surrounded by their bank accounts or latest gadgets. What they always want is close personal contact as they prepare to let go of life. This is what is valuable.

- You make legal wills to determine the distribution of your assets upon death. You take time to plan and execute a legal will. A legal will is made by your brain and is of no value until after your death. Legal wills do nothing to promote your health while you are alive, other than peace of mind regarding your assets. Even this can be contentious and cause deterioration of health.

- By contrast, a legacy is very valuable and can add years to your life. A legacy comes from your heart, and the real value is during your life. A legacy is a goal to live by.

- Knowing your legacy creates a focus. With focus, you achieve your objectives and live a richer life. Creating a legacy lightens the heart. This promotes balance and health. This is why it is more important to focus on a legacy rather than a legal will.

- Living your legacy gives you life as you fulfill it.

- If you make wise choices and are disciplined, you have a legacy that impacts others and in a positive way. The biggest impact of a legacy may be for yourself as you are alive. If you make poor choices and are passive, your legacy is limited and has little impact. Which would you rather have?

Obviously, most people want a rich legacy, but to get a rich legacy, you need to make active choices every day. A legacy need not be a document. However, you do have to take time to reflect and think about what you do want your legacy to truly be.

A true legacy changes every day with your actions, but at the same time is consistent with your greater vision.

- If you were to die suddenly today, would you be happy with your relationship with yourself, others, and a higher spirit?
- What would you want to be said at a memorial service for you, and how would you give your own eulogy?
- What issues do you need to resolve now so that you live your legacy while you are alive?

(This is your most important exercise for improved total relationships.)

Write in the space below your own legacy. Keep it brief and concentrate on what actions you do in your life. Pretend that you are at your own funeral and that you are going to give the eulogy. This may sound morbid, but it can be very important to the way you live today. Cultures that recognize death and even celebrate it do this to enhance their life and make them live with more intensity. Remember to live your legacy.

QUESTIONS TO IMPROVE YOUR RELATIONSHIPS

Journal your responses below: (you can use some of your previous responses in summary).

1. What do I need to do to remind myself that I am worthy? How can I serve others better so as to feel more worthy?

2. What do I need to do to be the type of person that I would like to be around? What trans-generational behaviors do I want to address?

3. How could I treat my friends and family in a more positive way?

4. What feelings and emotions do I need to express? Whom do I need to listen to more in life?

5. What are examples of how I have felt a higher spirit working in my life? What do I need to do to feel more of this?

6. What things in my life that I perceived as bad do I need to be grateful for?

7. Am I being the type of person that I want to be? Am I living the type of legacy that I want to leave when I die? Are my actions consistent with my desires?

CONCLUSION

Conclusion:

Making small, simple, positive, proactive changes through awareness can impact your life at any time. Break any robotic thinking you have with mindful choices.

Life by its nature is always changing. Being aware of that change and influencing what you can are the keys to improving your health.

Two final sayings to think about:

"Teach us to number our days so that we may gain a heart of wisdom" (adapted from Psalms 90:12).

Life is a wonderful gift. Each day is precious. Make the most of it, whatever your condition is, and SOAR.

"A heart at peace gives life to the body, so let this be your goal in life" (adapted from Proverbs 14:30).

As you gain peace in your own spiritual heart, this will be your greatest legacy. Peace comes through awareness.

PRESCRIPTION TO HELP YOU SOAR TO YOUR BEST POSSIBLE HEALTH

For_____ (your name here)

Cultivate daily **awareness** and take daily actions as follows:

- Cultivate **less** ungratefulness, hate, arrogance, and un-forgiveness in your brain.

- Cultivate **more** gratefulness, compassion, humility, and forgiveness in your heart.

- **Take care** of your physical body every day.

- Eat the way you want to **feel.**

- Mindfully **do** and express yourself every day so as to fulfill your purpose in life.

- **Be** the type of person you want to be.

Signed Dr. *Roger White*

(Access at your local Spiritual Heart Pharmacy)   (Unlimited Refills)

_____

FOR FURTHER INFORMATION REGARDING THE SOAR
TOTAL HEALTH IMPROVEMENT SEMINARS, GO TO
www.SOARtotalhealthimprovement.com